The Treasure of the Palms: The Dates

between history and legend,

between science and well-being

Codice ISBN: 9798305471151
Casa editrice: Independently published

To Giovanni, Natalina and Chanel, thank you for the love you have given me, we have never left each other.
You are always here close to me, in mind and heart.

Summary

Premise

The content of this book is taken exclusively from a reading and analysis of the scientific publications of the last decades that have concerned the date palm.

The fruit of the date palm (Phoenix dactylifera) has countless nutritional and nutraceutical properties that make it special compared to all other fruits. The purpose of the book is not to provide medical or nutritional information, for these needs you must contact your trusted doctor, instead the purpose is to make the Western public aware of the properties, history and legends of the date and bring people closer to this miraculous fruit that grows in territories with extreme climate, it is cultivated with ancient techniques but of current hydraulic engineering and, in these territories, represents an important economic aspect, but also particular cultural and religious aspects. Those who have the patience to read this book will discover stories and legends, biochemical properties and important uses in sport, gestation and childbirth, in neutralizing the effects of free radicals with its antioxidants and, more generally, the beneficial effects on the health of those who consume them in the right quantities.

Enjoy the reading

Marco Delledonne

Chapter 1: The Legend

The Song of the Palms

In a small village at the gates of the Moroccan desert, there lived a little girl named Amina. She was eight years old and had a smile that shone like the sun at dawn. Amina was the daughter of Ahmed and Fatima, two farmers who cultivated a small oasis of date palms, handed down from generation to generation.

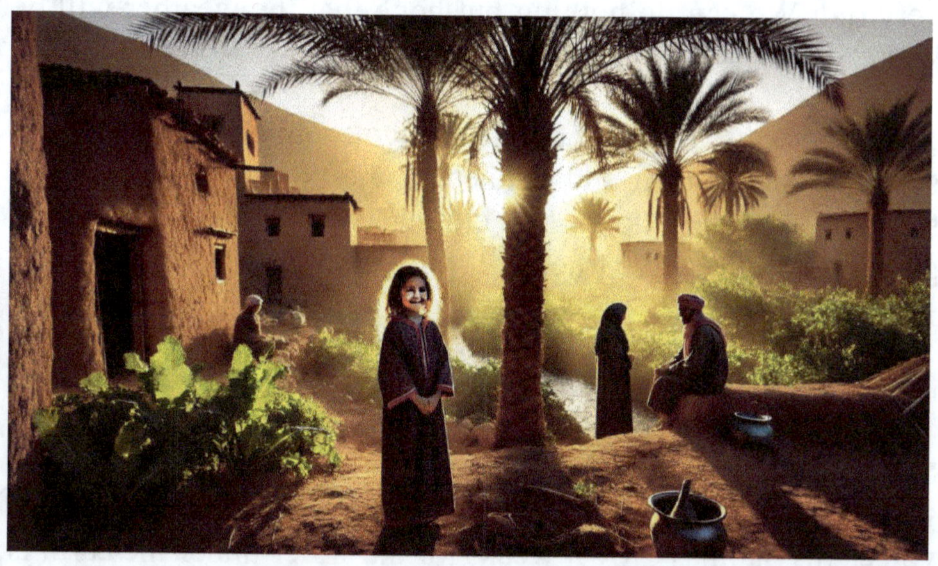

Every morning, before the sun got too hot, Amina woke up to help her parents. With small but agile hands, she collected the dates that had fallen to the ground and put them in baskets woven by her mother. She knew that every date was precious; not only for her family, but also for the merchants of the Erfoud market, who bought them to resell throughout the region.

One day, while picking the golden fruits, Amina noticed something strange: one of the palm trees, the oldest and tallest of all, seemed to wither. Its leaves were opaque and the dates fallen unripe. It was a special palm tree, called **Laila**, which her grandfather said was "the soul of the oasis".

"Dad," Amina said, pulling on Ahmed's tunic, "Laila is sick. We must help her!"

Ahmed sighed, stroking his daughter's head. "Amina, Laila is very old. We can do nothing but hope that the weather will be kind."

But Amina did not give up. That night, while the village was sleeping, she got up and walked to the palm tree. Under the starlight, she knelt down and closed her eyes, hoping that her grandfather tales were true.

'If you really have a soul,' she whispered to the palm tree, 'tell me how I can help you.'

Suddenly, a warm wind enveloped the air, and Amina heard a soft voice, like a whisper in the leaves. 'Little keeper,' said the voice, 'my sap has grown weak, for the water under the earth is scarce. But there is an ancient river hidden in the desert. Only the pure heart of a child can find it."

The next day, Amina told her parents about the dream. Ahmed laughed, thinking it was just fantasy, but Fatima looked at her with hopeful eyes. "Perhaps," said the mother, "grandfather legends were not just stories."

With a bottle of water and her small shepherd staff, Amina set off for the desert. The voice of the palm tree had told her to follow the song of the wind. She walked for hours, until the sun high in the sky seemed to melt everything. But when she was about to give up, she heard a sound: a melodious murmur, like a song dancing in the sand.

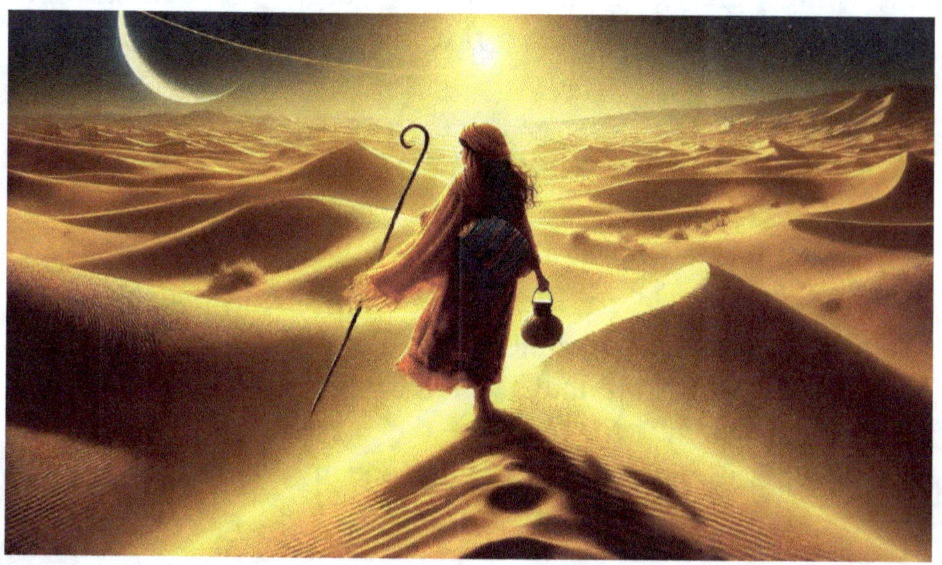

Following the sound, Amina came to a dune where she found a stone carved with ancient Berber symbols. 'Dig here,' said the wind. With her bare hands, he began to dig. The sand was hot and heavy, but Amina didn't stop. Finally, her fingers touched something damp: a small underground stream that shone like liquid silver.

She returned to the oasis with an amphora of pure water. She poured it around Laila's roots, singing a song her mother had taught her, an ancient hymn to life. Slowly, the palm tree seemed to awaken. Its leaves turned green again, and the dates became sweeter and more abundant than they had ever been.

From that day on, Amina's oasis flourished like never before. The market merchants began to call the dates "Golden Tears", so sweet were they. And every night, Amina returned to Laila, who now bent slightly to the wind, as if to embrace her, and told the palm tree about her dreams and adventures.

The village grew, but no one ever forgot the courage and goodness of Amina, the little girl who had listened to the singing of the palm trees.

The Children of the Desert

Under the blazing blue sky of Morocco, in the heart of a village on the edge of the desert, lived two brothers, Karim and his little sister Layla. Karim was nine years old, and Layla was seven; They were inseparable and found comfort in each other, even when life put them to the test. One day, a terrible fever took both their parents away, leaving them alone in the small mud and stone house where they were born.

After the funeral, an uncle, Ahmed, came from Tangier. He was a wealthy man with a generous heart. 'Come with me,' he said, 'I will give you a comfortable home and a better life.' But Karim shook his head, shaking Layla's hand. 'This is our home,' he said in a firm voice. "We cannot leave it."

The little house was not just a place; it was full of memories: the scent of mint tea prepared by their mother, the sound of the stories told by their father under the moon, and the company of their three inseparable friends: **Moussa**, the sand-furred cat; **Amira**, a sweet camel who gave them milk every morning; and **Zahra**, a lively goat who used to hop around the courtyard.

Karim and Layla decided to stay, but life was not easy. With little savings and no one to take care of them, they were forced to drop out of school. They found work on a date palm plantation run by poor but kind farmers. Their agility made them perfect for the job of tying nets around fruit-laden branches, so that the dates would not fall to the ground.

Every day they climbed the tall, swaying palm trees, their feather-light bodies dancing with the wind. The farmers treated them like children, bringing them warm bread and olives in their breaks and teaching them the art of palm care. Karim felt proud, protecting Layla with an adult determination.

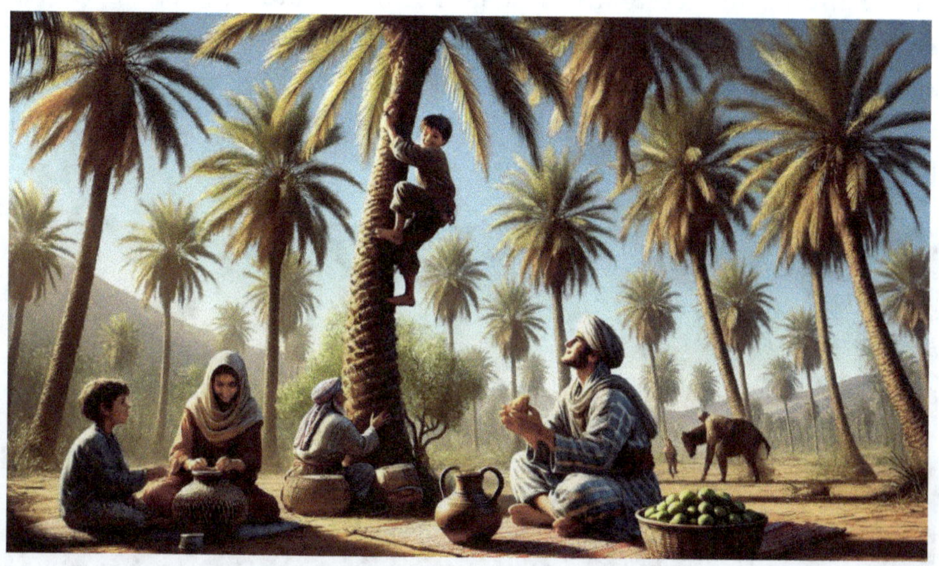

But one day, tragedy struck again. While standing on top of the plantation's tallest palm tree, Karim lost his balance. He fell heavily to the ground, and a heartbreaking cry filled the air. Layla ran to him, crying. The farmers took him home and called the village healer. "My back is hurt," he said the man, shaking his head. "He will no longer be able to walk as before."

Karim felt desperate, the weight of the world on his young shoulders. How could he take care of Layla? How could they survive? One night, as the wind blew through the palm branches, a voice woke him up. It was sweet and deep, like the whisper of an ancient spirit.

'Karim,' said the voice, 'I am Ahlam, the palm tree that saw you grow. Fear not. Earth always has a cure for those who love it. Eat twenty ripe dates in the morning and twenty in the evening. Do it for forty days, and your strength will return."

Karim thought it was just a dream, but the next day, he found under the palm tree a small basket full of golden dates, sweeter and juicier than any he had ever tasted. He decided to follow the advice of the voice. Every morning and evening, he counted twenty dates and ate them slowly, feeling a warm energy spread through his body.

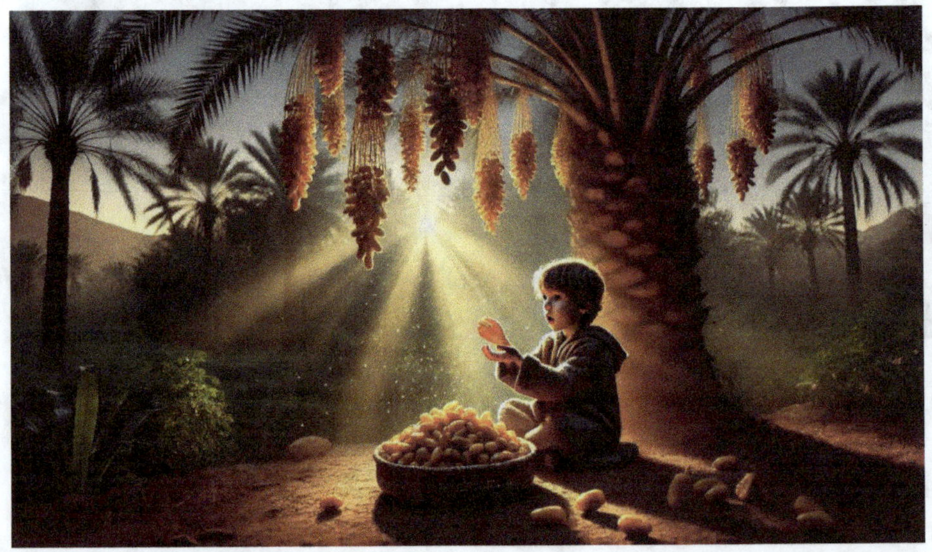

As the weeks passed, something miraculous happened. Karim began to feel a tingling sensation in his paralyzed leg. One day, he tried to move it and succeeded. Layla looked at him with wide eyes, full of hope. "You're healing, Karim!"

On the fortieth day, Karim got up. The leg was weak, but it worked again. He returned to the plantation, greeted by the smiles and tears of joy of the peasants. The story of the miracle spread throughout the village, and Karim became a symbol of hope and determination.

From that day on, the brothers continued to work, but they never stopped believing in the power of nature and the wisdom of the earth. Their home remained their refuge, a place of love and memories, where Moussa, Amira and Zahra waited for them every evening to tell them stories under the stars.

And every time Karim passed by the palm tree that had spoken to him, he stopped and caressed it. He knew that Ahlam was not just a tree, but an old soul, who would always protect them.

Chapter 2: The Cultivation of the Date Palm, an artificial ecosystem

The date palm (*Phoenix dactylifera L.*), belonging to the Arecaceae family, represents the pivotal species in the agricultural systems of the oases. Its importance lies both in its multiple uses and in the fundamental ecological role it plays in creating a favourable, often essential, environment for the cultivation of other species. The traditional date palm orchard is more than an agricultural system: it is a complex artificial ecosystem that reflects centuries of local knowledge and adaptation to the desert environment. The date palm, as a key species, not only feeds local communities but also supports biodiversity and ecological resilience in arid regions.

Date palms are also an iconic feature of the desert landscapes of North Africa and Southwest Asia. Like "islands of green" in seas of aridity, these oases mark the hot deserts, stretching from Morocco in the west to the Indo-Iranian borders in the east, and from central Syria in the north to Yemen in the south.

These are artificial, man-made ecosystems that defy the difficulties of a hostile environment and represent centres of agricultural productivity that also guarantee the subsistence of local populations. Despite their economic and symbolic importance both in the present and in the past, the origin and ancient history of these agro-systems still remain poorly understood.

Interdisciplinary studies indicate that the roots of agriculture in oases probably date back to prehistoric times, with a central area around the Persian Gulf.

Traditional date palm orchards are organized horizontally and vertically, with a tiered layout:

Upper Level:

Dominated by date palms, which can reach 20 meters in height. The large fronds provide shade to the plants below, protecting them from intense heat and reducing water evaporation.
Palm trees produce fruits rich in sugars, antioxidants, vitamins and mineral salts, but also other materials useful in the local economy:

1. **Stem and leaf veins**: Used for construction and fuel.
2. **Whole fronds**: Used for roofing or hut construction.
3. **Leaves**: Used for basketry, mats and ropes.
4. **Raw fibres (fibrillum)**: Suitable for ropes, baskets, packaging and padding.

Second Level:

Fruit trees of lower height grow under the palm trees, creating a diverse ecosystem.
The choice of species depends on local conditions, traditions and tastes. Fruit trees frequently grown in Middle Eastern palm gardens include:

1. **Fig** (*Ficus carica L.*).
2. **Pome granate** (*Punica granatum L.*).
3. **Thorn of Christ** (*Ziziphus spina-Christi* (L.) Desf.).
4. **Banana** (*Musa paradisiaca L.*).
5. **Mango** (*Mangifera indica L.*).
6. **Papaya** *L.*
7. **Citrus** fruits: Various species of oranges, lemons, and other fruits.

Orchards therefore represent:

1. **A resilient ecosystem**:
    - Vertical layering optimizes the use of sunlight, water, and soil resources.
    - The shade of palm trees reduces soil erosion and the risk of desertification.
2. **Local sustenance**:
    - Palm trees provide food, building materials, and everyday items.
    - Crop diversity ensures food security and income for local communities.
3. **Adaptation to extreme weather conditions**:
    - This agricultural model is an example of sustainability in arid environments, making the most of limited resources.

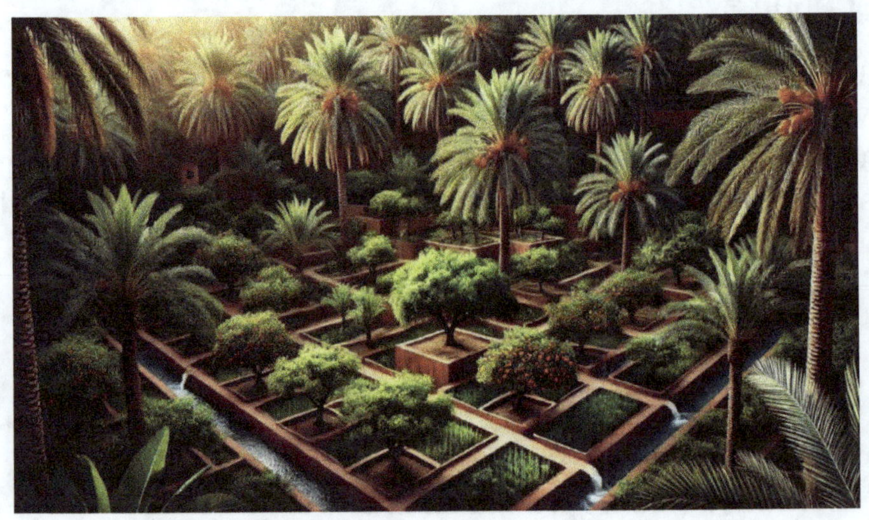

Chapter 3: History of Date Palms

Ancient Origins of the Date Palm

The date palm (*Phoenix dactylifera*) is one of the oldest cultivated plants in the history of mankind, dating back about 5,000 years.

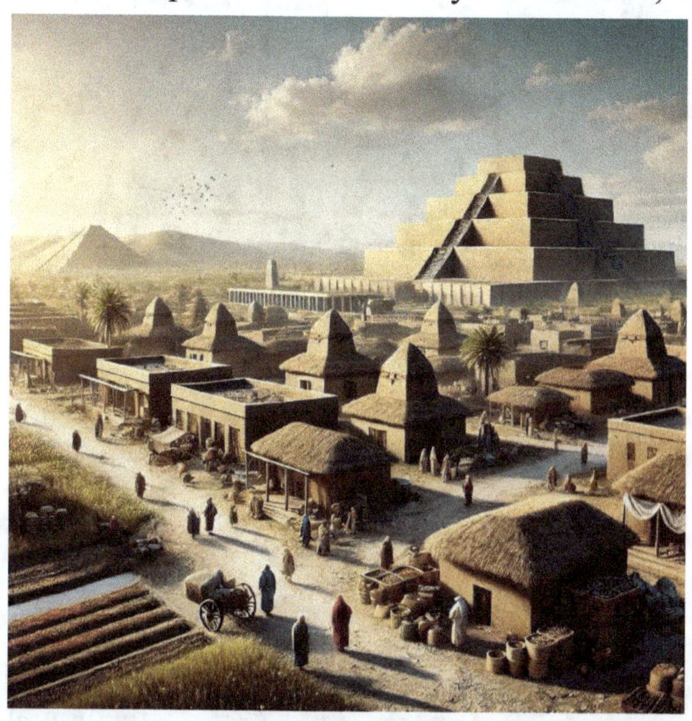

Native to Mesopotamia and the surrounding regions of the Persian Gulf, the date palm was a critical resource for ancient civilizations, providing food, building materials, and spiritual symbols. In Mesopotamia, the date was considered an essential food resource and a commodity, as documented in clay tablets written in cuneiform. Date palms were also symbols of fertility and prosperity, often depicted in Mesopotamian art and sculpture.

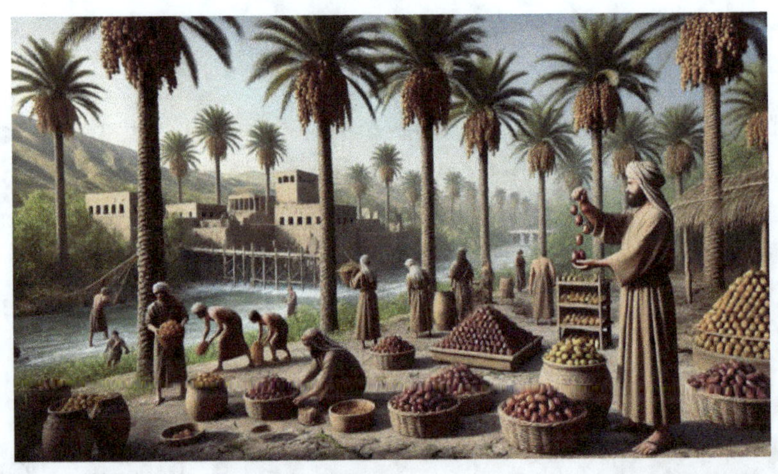

Mesopotamia and the Indus Valley: The first archaeological evidence indicates that the date palm was cultivated as early as 3,000 BC in the region between the Tigris and Euphrates. Dates were used for bartering and as a basic ingredient to prepare fermented drinks.

Ancient Egypt:

In ancient Egypt, dates were prized not only as a food, but also for ritual and medicinal purposes. They were included in funeral offerings to accompany the deceased to the

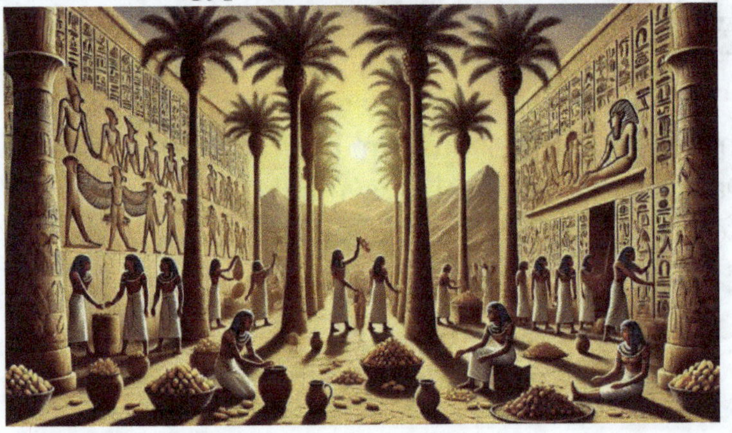

afterlife and used in the production of date wine. Hieroglyphics testify to the central role of the date in Egyptian agriculture, with representations of palm trees in the reliefs of the tombs.

Spread in the Mediterranean area: Commercial and cultural expansion brought date palms to North Africa, the Arabian Peninsula and later to southern Europe through Phoenician and Roman trade.

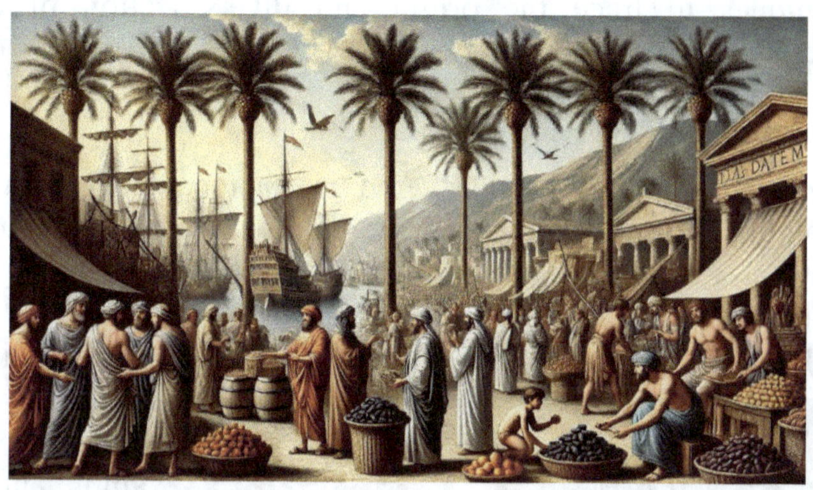

Archaeological evidence

Remains of dates have been found in archaeological sites in the Middle East and North Africa, confirming their cultivation and use since ancient times. Date seeds recovered from Egyptian tombs and sites of the Indus civilization testify to their spread along ancient trade routes. Scientific literature supports the centrality of the date in history and religion. Archaeobotanical studies, such as that of Zohary and Hopf (2000), highlight the early domestication of the date palm in Mesopotamia. Tengberg (2012) delved into the role of the date in the economy of ancient agricultural societies, demonstrating its importance as a food and commercial resource. Hawting (2003) and Nevo (1991) explore the symbolic and practical meaning of the date in religious contexts, especially in Judaism and Islam. Further research includes the analysis of date seed remains in archaeological contexts (Terral et al., 2012), which revealed information on the spread of date palm cultivation through trade routes. Recent studies by Murphy and Fuller (2017) have used genetic analysis techniques to trace the origin and diversification of date varieties.

The Palm as a Cultural and Religious Symbol

The date palm has been revered in many ancient cultures, becoming a symbol of prosperity and abundance. The date is mentioned in numerous religious and sacred texts, taking on symbolic and practical significance.

In the Old Testament, the date appears frequently, associated 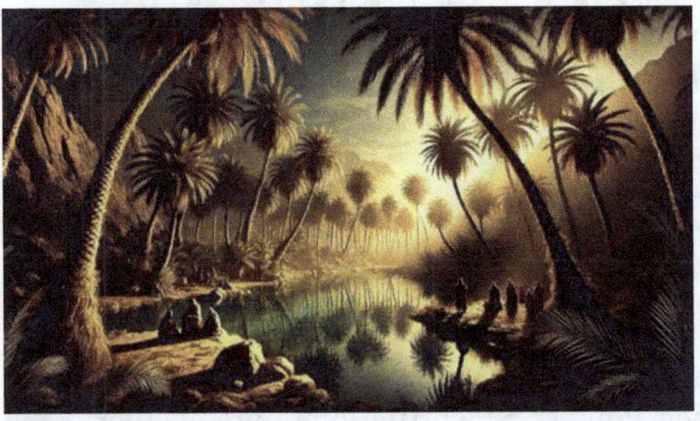 with fertility and abundance. For example, in the Book of Exodus, palm trees and dates are described as part of the landscape of the oasis of Elim (Exodus 15:27). Palm trees were considered symbols of victory and justice, as seen in the Psalms (Psalm 92:12).

Palm trees were considered symbols of victory and justice:

Salmi 92:12
"The righteous will blossom like the palm tree and grow like the cedar of Lebanon." Here the palm tree, from which dates are obtained, is a symbol of justice, longevity and beauty, representing the prosperity of those who live according to the divine will.

1 Re 6:29
"In the walls of the sanctuary, all around, both inside and outside, he carved figures of cherubs, palm trees and blooming flowers." Palm trees (reminiscent of dates) decorated Solomon's Temple, representing the beauty and abundance of God's Kingdom.

Deuteronomio 8:8
"It is a land of wheat, barley, vines, figs and pomegranates; it is a land of olive trees and honey."
Here "honey" could refer not only to bee honey, but also to the sweet date syrup, very common in the Jewish tradition.

Cantico dei Cantici 7:7-8
"Your stature resembles a palm tree and your breasts like its clusters. I said: I will climb the palm tree; I will gather the bunches of its fruits."
In this poetic passage, the palm tree and its fruits (dates) are symbols of beauty and fertility, linked to the figure of the beloved woman.

Levitico 23:40

"On the first day you will take fruit from the best trees, palm branches, branches of leafy trees and willows of the stream, and you will rejoice before the Lord your God for seven days."
During the festival of Sukkot (Festival of Tabernacles), palm branches, reminiscent of the oasis and dates, are an element of celebration and gratitude for divine protection.

In the Islamic world, dates are a sacred food. The Quran mentions the date in several passages, emphasizing its value nutritional and spiritual aspects. It is said that the Virgin Mary consumed dates during labour to gain strength and comfort (Surat Maryam, 19:23-26). In addition, the date is traditionally consumed to break the fast-during Ramadan, following the example of the Prophet Muhammad.

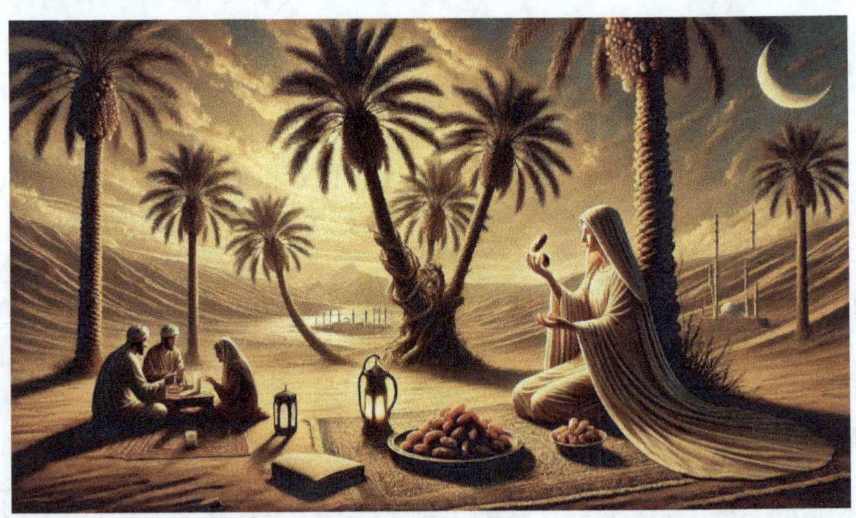

Vedic Texts and Other Traditions: Although less frequently mentioned, the date also appears in texts and traditions of other ancient cultures, such as the Indian one, where it was prized for its nourishing properties and its use in Ayurvedic medicine.

Mesopotamia and Babylon

In Mesopotamian civilizations, the palm tree was associated with fertility deities such as Ishtar. It represented abundance and the connection between heaven and earth. Sumerian texts, such as the myth of Inanna and Šukaletuda, tell of the creation of the palm tree by the god Enki, highlighting the importance attributed to this plant in local mythology.
The Babylonians used the trunks of palm trees to build houses and dates as a ritual offering.

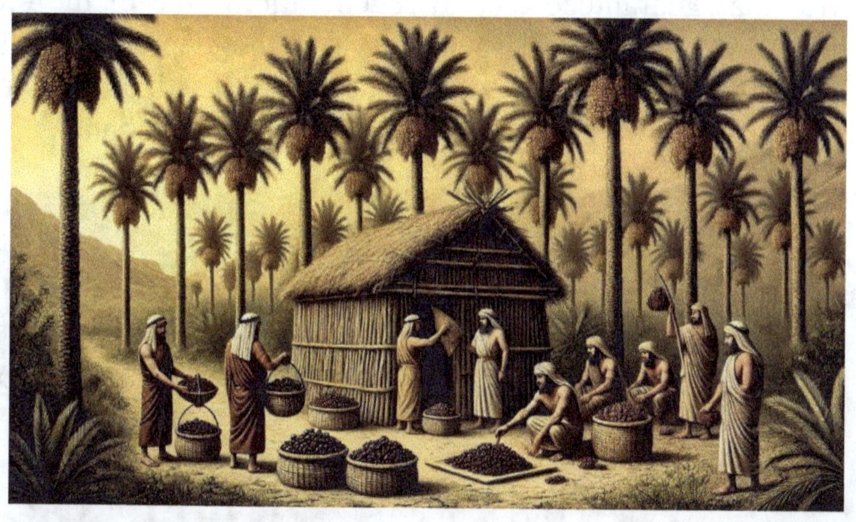

The date palm was widely cultivated in the plains of lower Mesopotamia. Its fruits, dates, were eaten fresh during the summer season, dried for the winter or processed into sweeteners through pressing. In addition, the leaves and sap of the trunk were used for food and craft purposes. Palm cultivation required specific techniques, such as manual pollination, which were labour-intensive. This practice contributed to the development of advanced agricultural skills in the region.

Ancient Egypt

In the complex religious symbolism of Ancient Egypt, the date palm was closely associated with the goddess Hathor, a central figure in Egyptian mythology. Hathor, goddess of fertility, joy, music and love, was also connected to the life cycle and regeneration. Hathor, often depicted as a woman with bovine horns enclosing a sun disk, was also seen as a celestial deity linked to rebirth. In his funerary role, Hathor welcomed the deceased into the realm of the afterlife, offering them the "water of life" that guaranteed eternal regeneration. One of the most iconic aspects of this association was the depiction of the goddess offering the "water of life" to the deceased, often placed on top of a palm tree, a symbol of renewal and abundance.

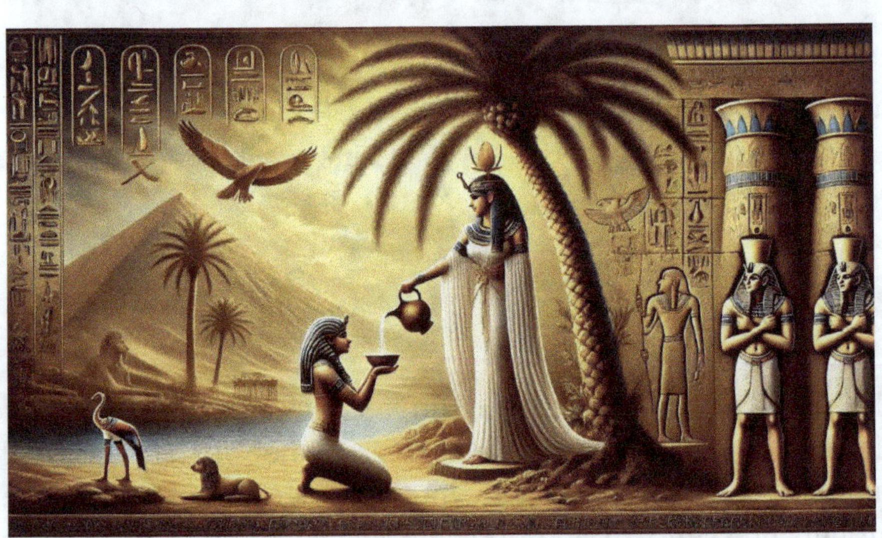

The god Thoth was also sometimes depicted counting the years on palm leaves, as it was believed that the tree produced a new leaf every month, and this symbolized the passage of time and eternity.

Thoth, often depicted as a man with the head of an ibis or

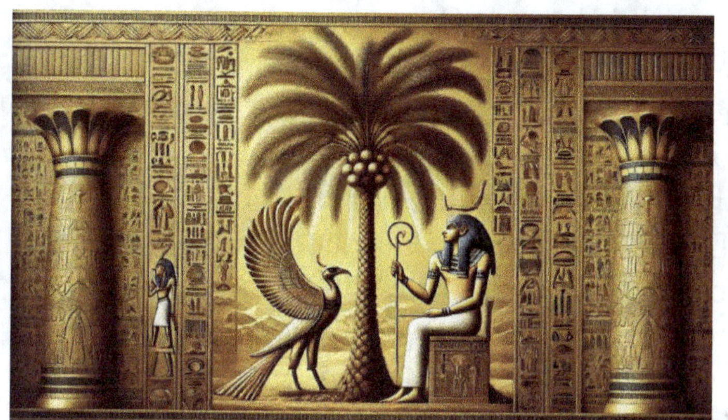

baboon, was the patron saint of the scribe and the inventor of hieroglyphics. He was also considered the keeper of time and the measurer of cosmic order. The importance of Thoth in the context of time is further reinforced by its association with the calendar. The month of Thoth ushered in the new year in the Egyptian calendar, an event marked by the arrival of the flooding of the Nile, a symbol of fertility and renewal. The use of palm leaves to count the years was a way to ground the abstract concept of time into a concrete and familiar symbol. In his function as controller of the calendar, Thoth was responsible for establishing the balance between the solar and lunar cycles, thus regulating the rhythms of human and natural life.

Time, in the Egyptian conception, was not just a linear entity, but an eternal cycle that reflected cosmic balance. Counting the years on palm leaves emphasized this cyclical view of time, as the palm tree itself was a symbol of regeneration. The palm tree was also a symbol of resurrection and immortality. During funeral ceremonies, palm branches were placed on the sarcophagi or on the chests of the mummies as a wish for the afterlife.

Greece and Rome

The ancient Greeks knew and appreciated the date palm, as attested by references in Homer's Odyssey.
Odissea, VI, 162-163
"I judge you like a young palm tree that I saw one day sprout near the altar of Apollo at Delos..."
When Odysseus meets Nausicaa, he compares her to a palm tree he once saw at Delos, near the sanctuary of Apollo. Odysseus compares Nausicaa to the young palm tree, highlighting her beauty, grace and purity. The young palm represents natural perfection and admiration for something extraordinary. The image of the palm tree near the sanctuary of Apollo reinforces the sense of sacredness and respect that Odysseus feels for the princess. The palm tree is seen as a special tree, often associated with the divine and sacred places. The palm tree, in the Mediterranean context, also symbolizes life and fertility, themes closely connected to the figure of Nausicaa, a young woman of marriageable age, and to the renewal that the hero hopes to find after his long journey.
The Greeks called the palm tree "phoinix," a meaningful term that reflects both the connection to the natural world and the cultural influences of the ancient Mediterranean. This name could be the origin of the modern scientific term, which combines "Phoenix" with "dactylifera" (from the Greek "dàktylos", finger, for the shape of the fruit).
The term "phoinix" has several possible origins and interpretations:
1.   The link with the Phoenicians: The word may derive from the Phoenician people (Phoinikes), known for their trade in the

Mediterranean, including the spread of the date palm. Palm trees were characteristic of the regions colonized by the Phoenicians and their trade routes.

2.   The colour purple: "Phoinix" in Greek also means "purple red" or "scarlet", referring to the colour of the ripe fruits of the palm tree or the legendary Phoenix bird, associated with rebirth. In Greek culture, the palm tree occupied a prominent place as a symbol of victory and triumph, a recurring image in celebrations related to sporting, military and divine achievements. This bond is further strengthened thanks to the figure of the goddess Nike, winged goddess of victory, often represented with a palm frond or a crown, emblems of success and honour. Often depicted flying to award winners, Nike carried a palm frond in her right hand, symbolizing divine recognition of their triumph.

The association of the palm tree with triumph has deep roots in Greek culture. This tree, with its majestic appearance and its ability to regenerate even in harsh environments, was seen as a natural symbol of resilience and success. Palm fronds were used to reward winners in Panhellenic games, such as the Olympic Games, where they were delivered along with other rewards, such as olive wreaths or laurel. Receiving a palm meant not only being recognized as a winner but also being celebrated as heroes worthy of glory.

In the Roman Empire, palm trees were associated with victory and triumph, used to celebrate military conquests.

In the Roman military context, the palm tree represented the triumph par excellence. During triumph celebrations, an honour bestowed on victorious generals, palms were carried in procession as tangible signs of victory. Victorious soldiers and commanders were often depicted holding palm fronds or receiving crowns intertwined with palm leaves, testifying to their success.

An important testimony of the association between the palm tree and victory can be found in Roman coins. Effigies of victorious emperors were often accompanied by images of palm trees, sometimes in the company of the goddess Victoria (the Roman equivalent of Nike). These coins served as propaganda tools, celebrating military achievements and reinforcing the image of imperial power in the eyes of the people.

The palm tree symbolized not only physical victory over enemies, but also the Roman order's assertion over chaos. In this sense, the tree was a symbol of the power and stability of the Empire.

The Romans consumed both fresh and dried dates, using them in confectionery preparations and to flavour wine. In addition, an alcoholic beverage was obtained from the fermentation of dates. The palm tree was a symbol of victory and triumph in Roman culture as well. Victorious gladiators received a palm branch in recognition of their success.

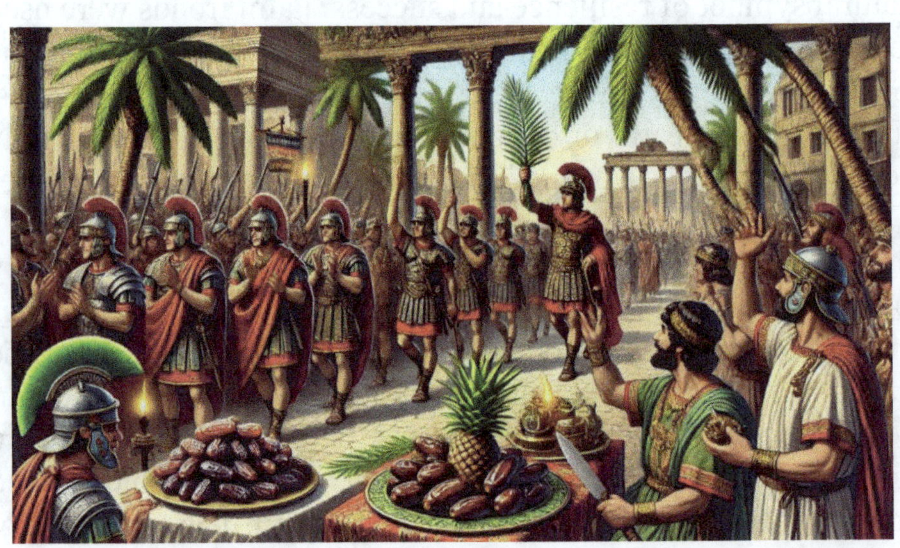

The palm tree in Islamic and Medieval History

With the advent of Islam in the seventh century, the date palm (Phoenix dactylifera) took on a deeply spiritual and cultural significance, becoming a central symbol in the religion and daily life of Muslims. Already venerated for its nutritional and economic value in pre-Islamic desert societies, the palm tree was further sacralised through the Qur'an and prophetic tradition, becoming an emblem of blessing, resilience and divine generosity.

Islamic References

The palm tree is mentioned numerous times in the Qur'an, highlighting its importance as a divine gift. The Prophet Muhammad (peace be upon him) encouraged the consumption of dates and considered them a blessed food, particularly during the month of Ramadan. Even in the hadith (sayings of the Prophet Muhammad), the palm tree is praised for its spiritual and practical value. Muhammad calls it "the blessed tree" and compares it to the faithful believer, as both are solid, productive, and full of virtue. This comparison highlights the ethical qualities that Muslims should emulate: resilience in difficulties, generosity, and usefulness to the community.

Agricultural expansion

During the medieval period, palm cultivation techniques were perfected by the Arabs, who introduced advanced irrigation to "qanat" to maximize yield.
Medieval Arab agronomists and farmers developed advanced knowledge about the date palm, thanks to their first-hand experience in the countries of the Middle East and North Africa. Key innovations include:

Irrigation Techniques: The Arabs perfected irrigation systems such as qanats (underground canals) and sakieh (water wheels),

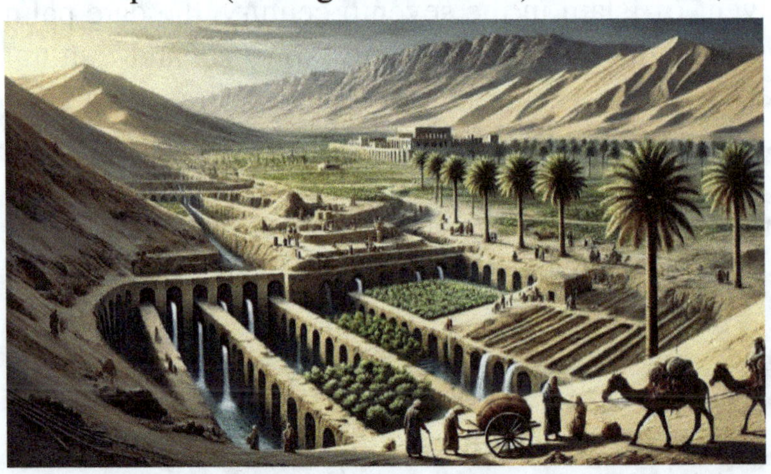

which allowed water to be brought to the driest oases. These systems were critical to ensuring the survival of palm trees, which require a lot of water to grow in extremely hot climates.

- Variety Selection: Arab agronomists introduced methods to select the most resistant and productive palm varieties, adapting them to different microclimates. This genetic improvement led to the spread of fine varieties, some of which are still considered among the best in the world, such as the Deglet Nour.
- Propagation techniques: The Arabs perfected the art of propagation through suckers (basal shoots), which made it possible to obtain plants genetically identical to mother palms, ensuring a constant quality of the fruits.

With the Islamic conquests, the date palm spread to Spain, where it thrived thanks to the symbiosis between Arab techniques and the Mediterranean climate. In Spain it was the caliph Abdurrahman I who in 756 AD was the first to plant specimens in Cordoba in his garden.

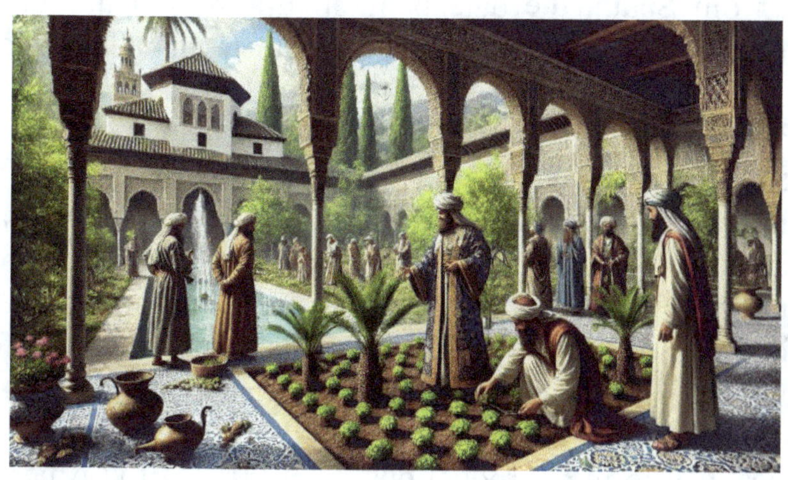

The "Palm Grove of Elche", declared a UNESCO World Heritage Site for its beauty, is in Spain in the province of Alicante and consists of more than half a million palm trees that make it the largest palm grove in Europe, surpassed in the world only by a few Arab palm groves.

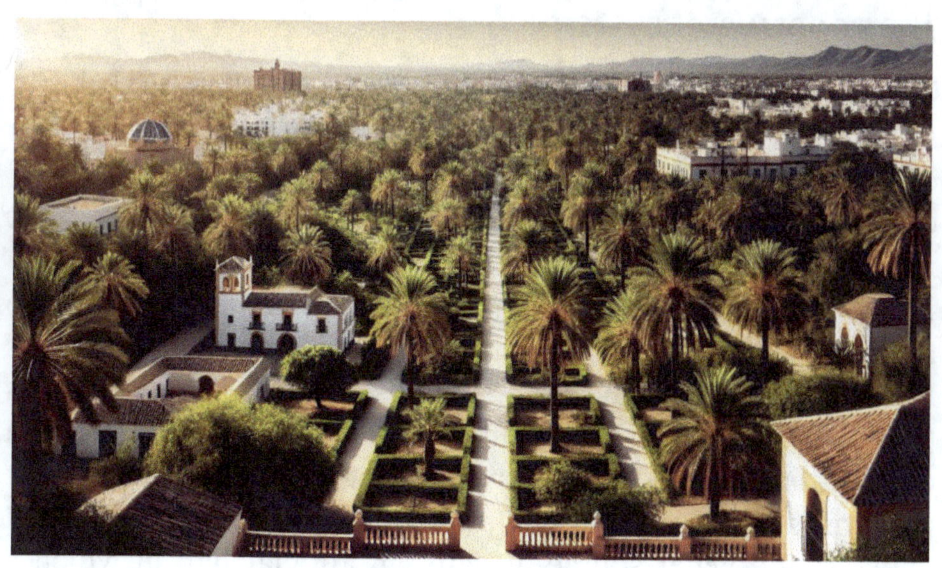

Apart from Spain, the date palm in Europe remains only an ornamental plant that due to the climate is unable to ripen its fruits. The date palm was also introduced in 1869 in North India and Pakistan, not numerous cultivations of date palms are even found in Australia.

The spread in the Americas is instead due to the Spanish Missionaries who introduced them in Mexico and California starting in 1765. Since the end of the 1800s, cultivation in California has become intensive with the cultivation of different varieties of dates. Today the cultivation can count on 6000-7000 hectares cultivated with date palms of the highest quality varieties. Californian productions meet 90% of the Americans' date needs, while Arab countries hold the top positions in date production. Around 5 million tons of dates are produced worldwide per year. Egypt is the first exporting country of this food, reaching a production of about 1,500,000 tons of dates per year, followed by Iran and Saudi Arabia.

The qanat water system

Throughout the arid regions of Iran, agricultural and permanent settlements are supported by the ancient qanat system that exploits the alluvial aquifers at the head of the valleys and conducts water down underground tunnels by gravity, often for many kilometres. The eleven qanats that represent this system include rest areas for workers, water tanks and water mills. The traditional municipal management system still in place allows for fair and sustainable sharing and distribution of water. Qanats provide an exceptional testimony to cultural traditions and civilizations in desert areas with an arid climate. Each qanat comprises a nearly horizontal tunnel that collects water from an underground water source, usually an alluvial fan, in which a mother well is dug at the appropriate level of the aquifer. Shaft wells are dug at regular intervals along the tunnel route to allow for the removal of waste material and allow ventilation. These appear as craters from above, following the line of the qanat from the water source to the agricultural settlement. The water is transported along underground tunnels, the so-called koshkan, by gravity due to the gentle slope of the tunnel to the exit (mazhar), from where it is distributed via canals to the farmers' farmland.

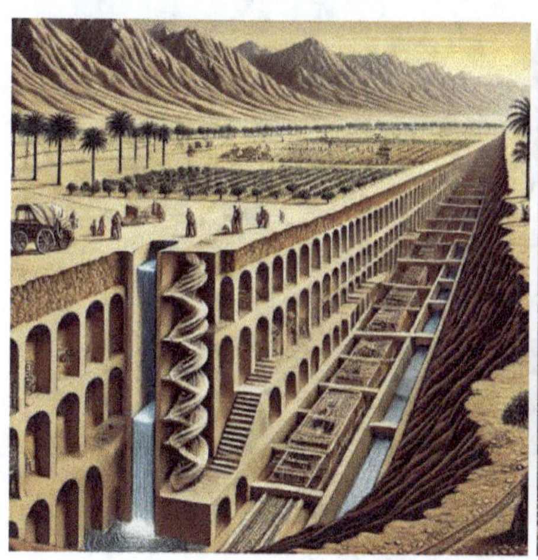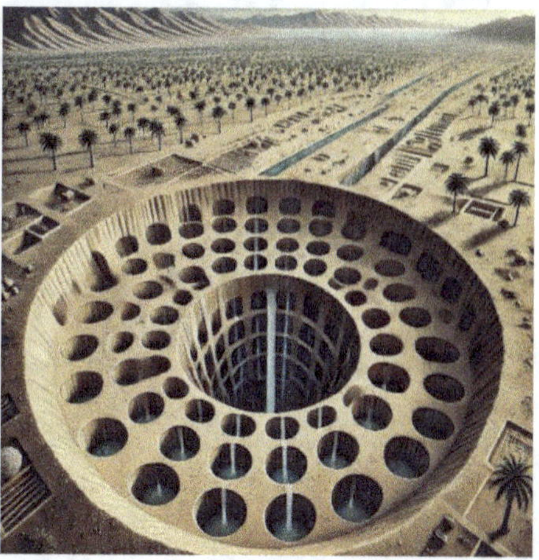

Global Economy

Dates are a multibillion-dollar industry, with growing demand in Europe, Asia, and North America. Exports have made dates accessible around the world, transforming them from a traditional food to a global product.

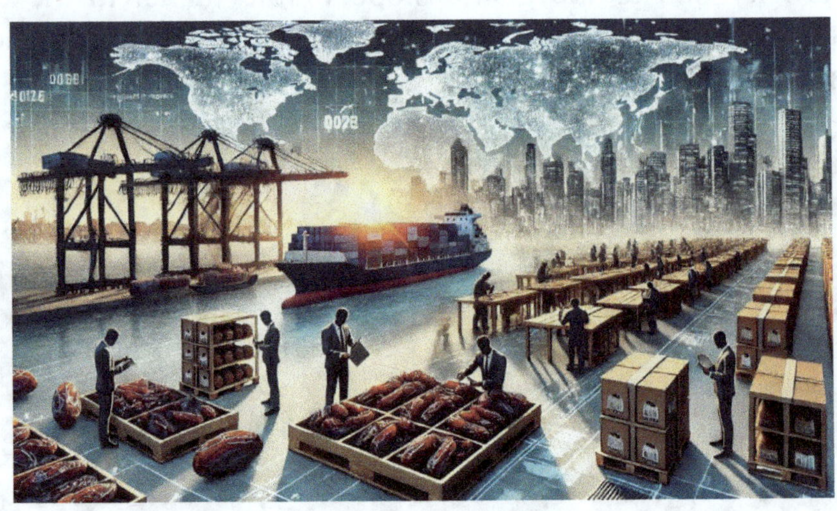

The main date-producing countries include Saudi Arabia, Egypt, Iran and the United Arab Emirates, which dominate the global scene in terms of both quantity produced and exports. Egypt alone produces about a fifth of the world's dates, while countries such as Iraq and Saudi Arabia offer renowned varieties, such as Deglet Nour and Medjool, which are particularly popular in international markets. Modern cultivation, processing and storage techniques have made it possible to increase yields and improve fruit quality, thus responding to growing demand. Investments in technology and infrastructure have transformed the date industry into an increasingly sophisticated industry. In recent decades, date consumption has grown significantly in

Europe, Asia, and North America. This increase in demand is due to several factors:

- Health trends: Dates, rich in fibre, vitamins, minerals and natural sugars, are increasingly popular as a healthy snack and source of energy. Their low-fat content and total absence of cholesterol make them a natural alternative to industrial snacks.
- International Cuisine: The spread of Middle Eastern and North African cuisine has introduced dates as a versatile ingredient in sweet and Savory dishes. In addition, dates are used in the preparation of innovative products such as energy bars, natural sweeteners and spreads.
- Seasonal and Religious Demand: The demand for dates increases particularly during Ramadan, when they are traditionally consumed to break the fast, but also during the holiday season and other cultural events, reflecting their spread on a global scale.

Chapter 4: The Qur'an and Dates

The Qur'an is the sacred text of Islam, considered by Muslims to be the word of God (Allah) revealed to the Prophet Muhammad through the archangel Gabriel (Jibril). The Qur'an is not only a book of religious doctrine, but a literary masterpiece and a pillar of Islamic culture. Its form, structure and presentation reflect its sacredness and its profound meaning for believers. The term derives from the Arabic al-Qur'an, which according to some scholars is of Syriac derivation and is to be linked to the verb qara'a, "to read". The Qur'an is therefore a reading aloud, a recitation. The Qur'an consists of 114 chapters, called suras (Arabic: سورة), which vary in length from a few verses (ayat) to hundreds. The suras are organized in descending order of length, with some exceptions, and do not follow a chronological order of revelation. Each surah has a title that usually comes from a significant word or theme present in the chapter, such as Al-Baqara ("The Heifer") or An-Nur ("The Light"). The individual verses, called ayat (Arabic: آيات, "signs"), are numbered and represent the fundamental units of the text. In total, the Quran contains about 6,236 verses, although the exact number may vary slightly depending on the recitation traditions.

The Content of the Qur'an is generally divided into three large parts: the precepts, the stories and exhortations, and the admonitions. To make it easier to read and memorize, the Quran is divided into smaller sections:

- Juz': The entire text is divided into 30 parts, called juz' (Arabic: جزء), to allow for a complete daily reading in a month, especially during Ramadan.
- Hizb: Each juz' is further divided into two hizb, creating 60 sections overall.

- Rukū': These are short thematic passages used in prayer and recitation.

The Quran is written in classical Arabic, which is considered the purest and noblest form of the Arabic language. It is appreciated for its rhythmic structure and stylistic richness, which make recitation (tilawah) a deeply spiritual practice. Some standout features include:

- Introduction with the Basmalah: Each surah (except one) begins with the formula "Bismillah ar-Rahman ar-Rahim" ("In the name of Allah, the Merciful, the Most Compassionate").
- Rhyming Text: Many ayats feature a rhythmic cadence, making it easier to memorize and act.
- Decorative calligraphy: Quran manuscripts are traditionally decorated with beautiful miniatures and ornaments, and Arabic calligraphy takes on a central artistic role.

Historically, the Quran was transcribed on various materials, from parchment sheets to wooden tablets, before being collected in book form (mushaf). The first mushaf were written in the Kufi style, characterized by angular and straight lines, while in later centuries more elaborate styles developed, such as Naskh and Thuluth. Today, the Qur'an is printed in millions of copies, respecting strict transcription rules to preserve the accuracy of the sacred text. Each edition must faithfully follow the rules of spelling and acting (tajweed), ensuring uniformity throughout the Islamic world.

Dates occupy a special place in the Qur'an and Islamic tradition, so much so that they are considered a symbol of blessing, nourishment and divine protection.

This chapter explores references to dates in the Quran, their spiritual significance, and some fantastic stories surrounding the date palm, interweaving faith and myth.

References to Dates in the Qur'an

The Qur'an mentions dates in numerous suras and verses, emphasizing their value as blessed food and a divine gift. Here are some significant examples:

Sura 2, verse 266 - Al-Baqarah (The Heifer) 2:266

"Would any of you have a garden of palm trees and vines, under

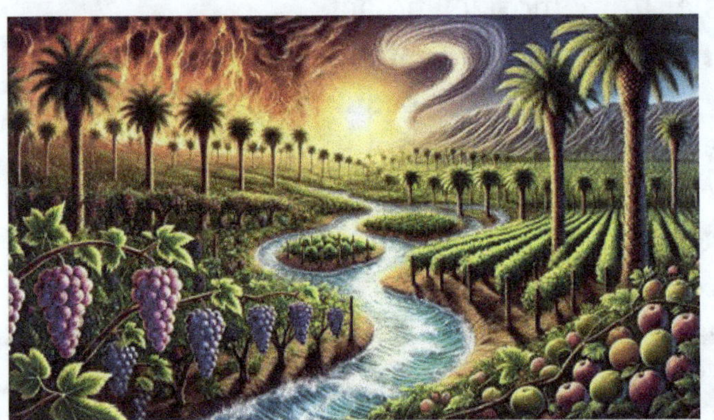

which streams flow, and give him all sorts of fruits, while he is seized by old age and his children are weak, and that he is struck with a whirlwind with fire, that burns him? So, Allah exposes His signs to you so that you can reflect."

This verse is a metaphor that invites believers to reflect on the importance of their actions and intentions. The garden represents the good works that an individual cultivates throughout his life. However, if these actions are not supported by sincere faith and good intentions, they risk being destroyed, like a garden struck by a whirlwind of fire.

Sura 6, verse 99 - Al-An'am (The Livestock) 6:99

"He is the One who brings down water from heaven. With it we

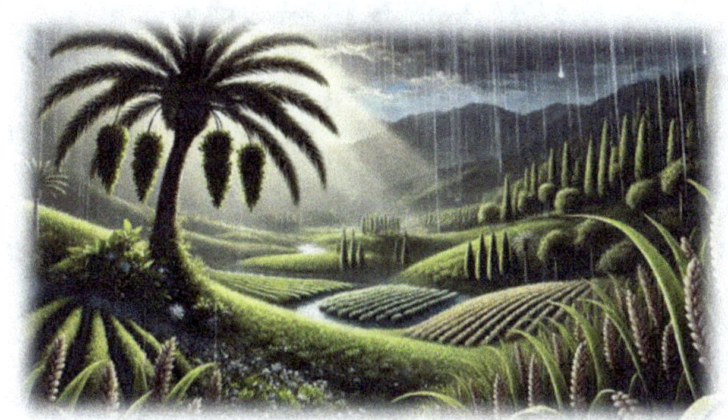

sprout all sorts of plants, from them we sprout vegetables and grains arranged in ears, and from the date palm, from its shoots, bunches of hanging dates ..."

This verse describes the cycle of plant life as a sign of divine power.

Sura 16, verse 11 - An-Nahl (Bees) 16:11

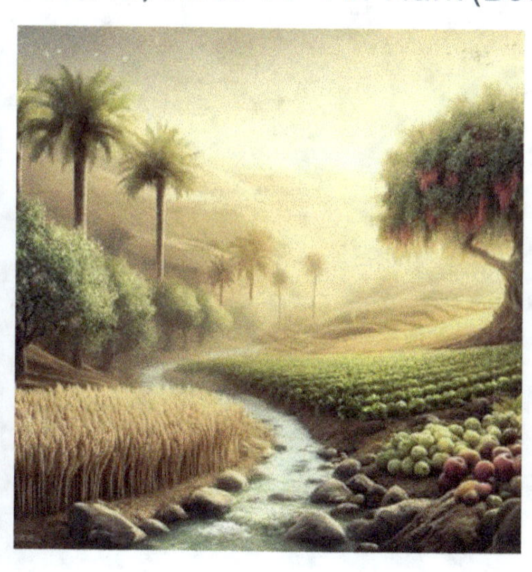

"With it [the water] makes cereals, olive trees, palm trees, vineyards, and all sorts of fruits grow for you. Here is a sign for those who reflect."

"And from the fruits of the palm trees and vines obtained drink

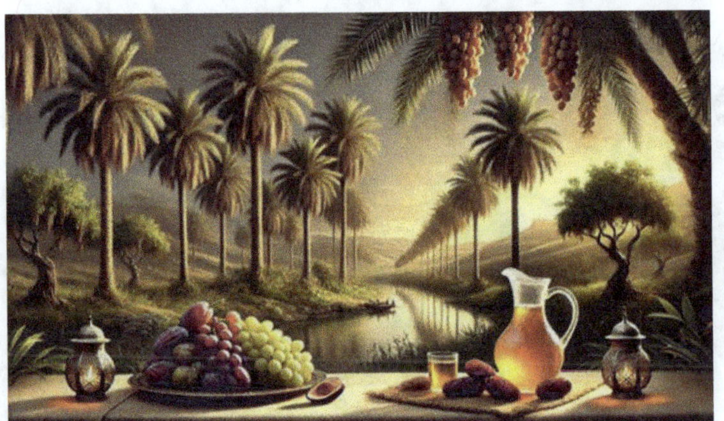

and good nourishment. Certainly, in this there is a sign for a people that understands."

Dates are praised here for their versatility and nutritional value, highlighting the link between food and spiritual reflection.

This passage tells the story of Mary (Maryam), the mother of Jesus, during childbirth:

"And the labour pains drove her toward the trunk of a palm

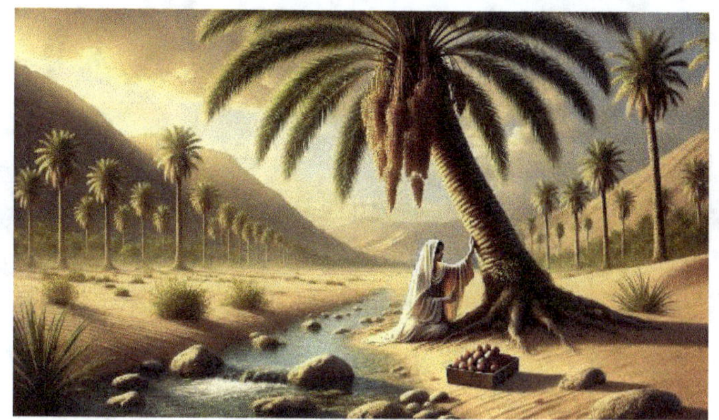

tree. She said, 'Oh, if I had died before this and been completely forgotten!'" (19:23)

"Then [the angel] called to her from under her: 'Do not grieve! Your Lord has set a stream at your feet and shake the trunk of the palm tree towards you: you will cause fresh and ripe dates to fall on you.'" (19:24-25)

Eat, drink, and be quiet..." (19:26)

Here the date is presented as a divinely provided food, with restorative properties during a time of great difficulty.

Sura 23, verse 19 - Al-Mu'minun (The Believers) 23:19

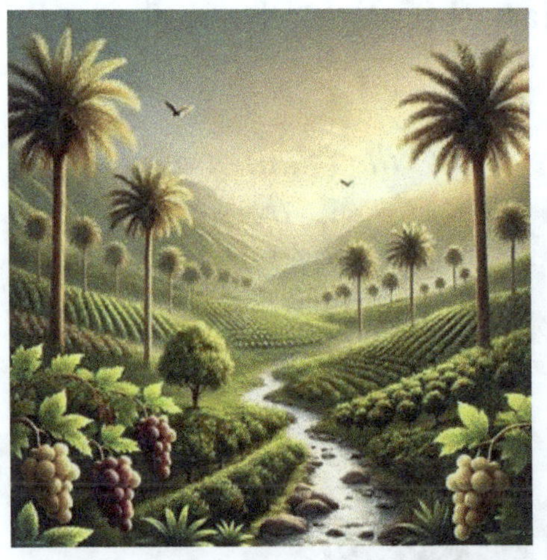

"And with it We made gardens of palm trees and vineyards sprout for you, in which you have abundant fruit and on which you are nourished."

The verse invites believers to reflect on the blessings they receive and to recognize Allah's generosity. Nature and its fruits are divine signs, demonstrating the perfection of creation and reminding us of the importance of gratitude to the Creator. In a broader context, this verse is part of the narrative of Surah Al-Mu'minun, which calls attention to the qualities of true believers and evidence of God's presence in creation.

Sura 36, verse 34 - Ya-Sin 36:34

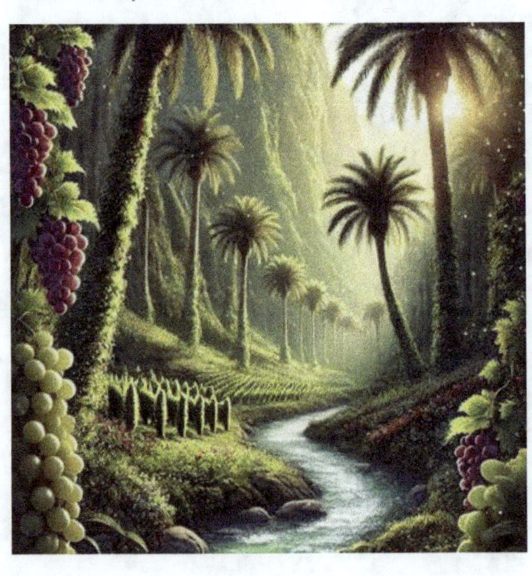

"And we have created in it gardens of palm trees and vineyards, and we have caused springs to spring up in it, "

The verse invites believers to reflect on the perfection and generosity of creation.

Gardens and springs are not only material resources, but also clear signs of Allah's mercy. Recognizing these blessings prompts gratitude and awareness of human dependence on the Creator.

Sura 50, verse 10-11 Qaf 50:10-11

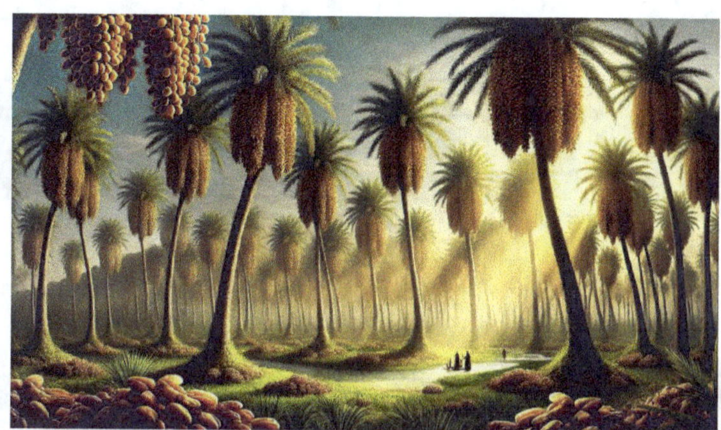

"And the slender palms with rich and overlapping clusters, nourishment for the servants."

Here the importance of dates as a source of sustenance for humanity is highlighted, a tangible sign of divine mercy.

Sura 55, verse 10-11 - Ar-Rahman (The Compassionate) 55:10

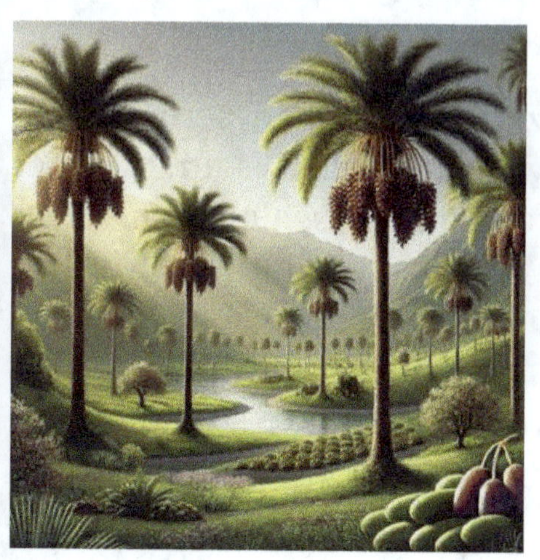

"And the earth has established it for creatures: in it are fruits and palms with protected spathes"

The verses invite gratitude to Allah for the land and its resources. The mention of palm trees emphasizes their importance both as a source of nourishment and as an example of divine generosity. The protected swords symbolize the care and order with which Allah manages creation.

Sura 80, verse 27-29 – Abasa 80:27-29

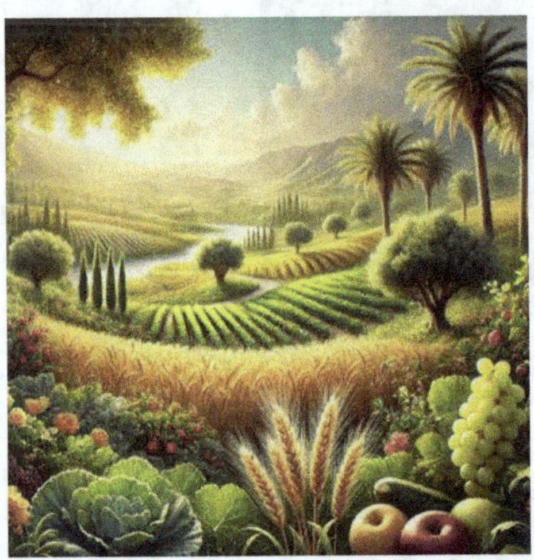

"And we sprout wheat, vines and vegetables, olive trees and palm trees..."

The verse invites us to recognize the order and perfection of divine creation, emphasizing how each element is arranged for the benefit of man. The mention of palm trees, along with other natural resources, reinforces the message of gratitude to Allah for life-sustaining gifts.

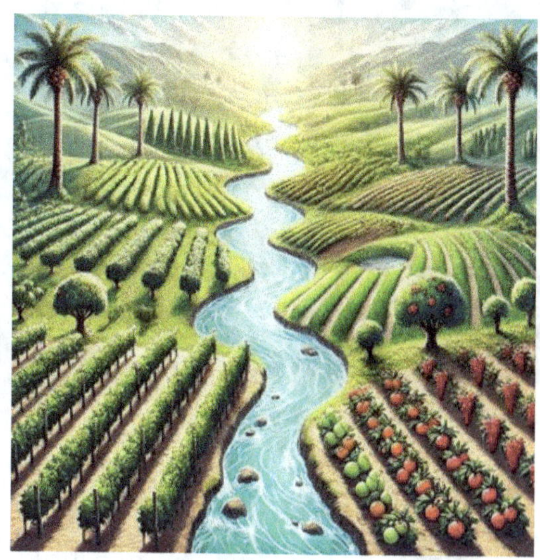

"On the land there are contiguous plots, vineyards and crops, palms grouped and isolated, watered by the same water. We favor some fruits over others."

The verse invites us to reflect on the wisdom and power of Allah, who has created an extraordinary variety of natural products for the benefit of humanity.

Every detail is a sign of His control and mercy, an invitation for believers to recognize His greatness.

Surat Ya-Sin (36:34-35)

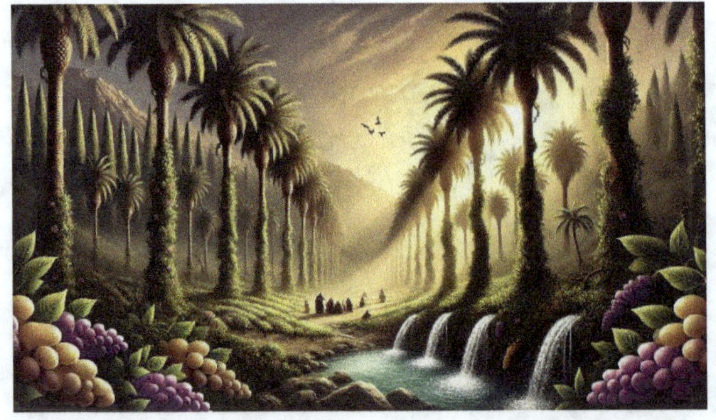

"And we have set up gardens of palm trees and vines in it, and have brought springs out of it, that they may eat its fruit and that which their hands have not produced."

Sura 78, verse 15-16 - An-Naba 78:15-16

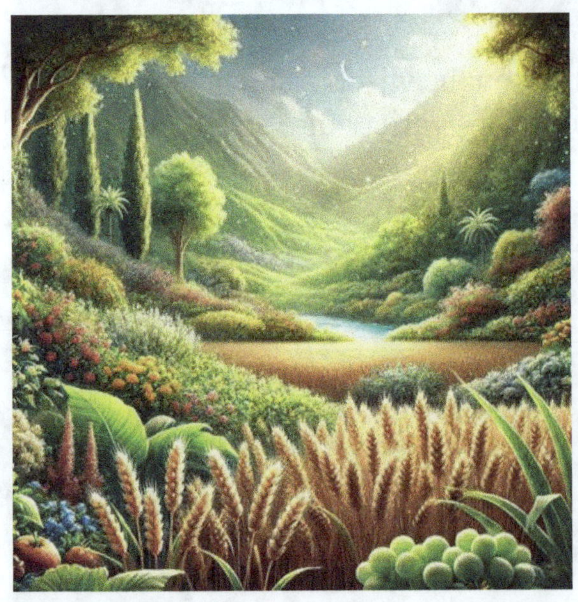

"That we may make cereals and plants sprout, and lush gardens."

Although he does not specifically mention dates, the reference to lush gardens may include date palms, given their centrality in Arab culture.

These verses invite believers to reflect on the perfection of Allah's creation and the fundamental role of nature as a means of sustenance and beauty. The emphasize the need to recognize and appreciate the blessings that come from this harmony.

Spiritual Significance and Islamic Tradition

The date in the Ramadan fast

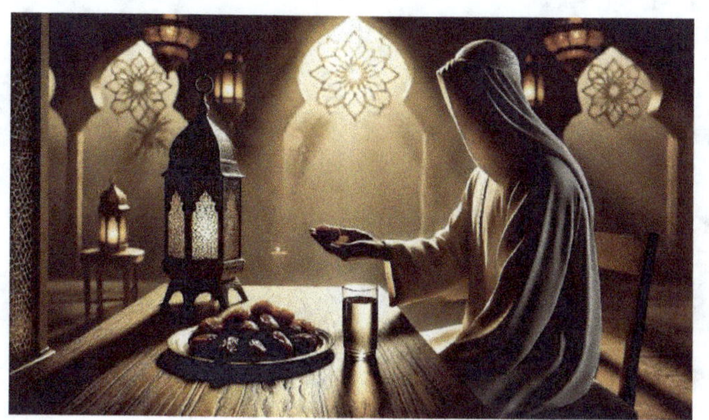

The date plays a central role in the fast of Ramadan, the holy month for Muslims during which fasting is practiced from dawn to dusk. The Prophet Muhammad (peace be upon him) recommended breaking the fast with dates, as recorded in several hadiths:

"When one of you breaks the fast, let him do it with a date, for it is a blessing; if he does not find a date, then with water, for it is pure." (Sunan Abu Dawood, 2356)

This practice, known as iftar, refers to the simplicity and spirituality of the prophetic gesture. Breaking the fast with a date recalls humility and gratitude to Allah for His blessings.

Dates as spiritual protection

According to a hadith (saying of the Prophet), eating seven Ajwa dates in the morning protects against poisons and evil influences.

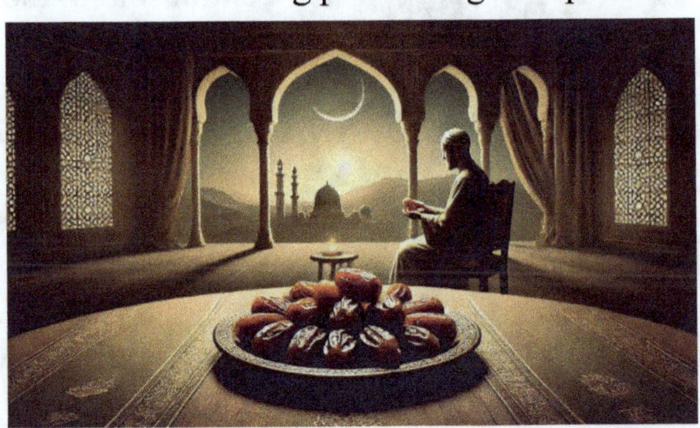

This reinforces the idea that dates are not only a food, but also a means of divine protection.

The date as a gift and charity

A food deeply rooted in Islamic culture, dates more than just sustenance. The Prophet Muhammad (peace be upon him) recommended giving dates to those in need, emphasizing their role in fighting hunger and promoting core values such as solidarity, generosity, and equality.

In the desert of the Arabian Peninsula, the date was one of the main sources of nutrition. Rich in sugar, fibre and minerals, it was considered a precious gift for relieving hunger and providing immediate energy. For this reason, the Prophet Muhammad encouraged his followers to share dates with those in need, remembering that even a simple gesture could have a great impact.

As recorded in one hadith:

"Protect yourselves from Hell, even if you donate only half a date to charity." (Sahih al-Bukhari, 1417).

This phrase shows that it is not the quantity of the gift that is important, but the sincere intention and desire to alleviate the suffering of others. Donating dates was not only a gesture of material generosity, but also a spiritual act. The Prophet Muhammad taught that every act of charity, no matter how small, brought the believer closer to Allah. The date, in its simplicity and abundance, represented the possibility for anyone to perform a meritorious action, regardless of their economic condition. This tradition of sharing dates has spanned the centuries and is still practiced in Islamic societies today, especially during Ramadan. Dates are distributed in mosques, markets, and homes, perpetuating the prophetic teaching that the well-being of a community is measured by the ability of its members to care for one another.

Fantastic Stories and Legends About Dates

Date palms are not only a source of religious inspiration, but also the protagonists of legendary tales handed down for generations.

The birth of the first palm tree

It is said that the first date palm was created from a handful of clay that was left over after the creation of Adam. God, seeing

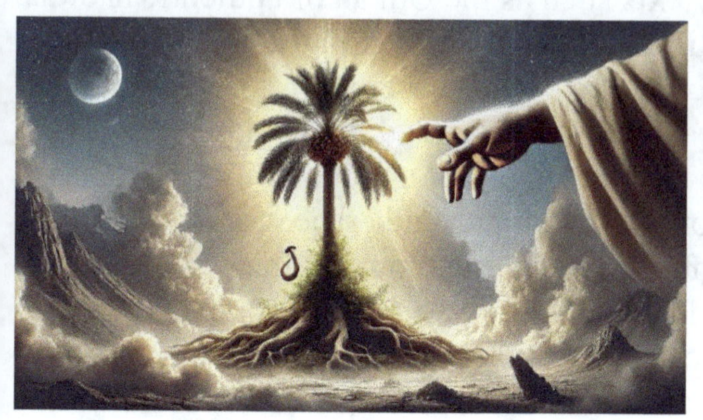

the beauty of the residual clay, fashioned a tree that would be a symbol of life and eternal nourishment for mankind. This legend attributes palm trees a direct link to the origin of life itself.

The Walking Palm

An ancient desert legend tells of a palm tree that moved at night to find water. It is said that, when the palm tree reached an oasis, 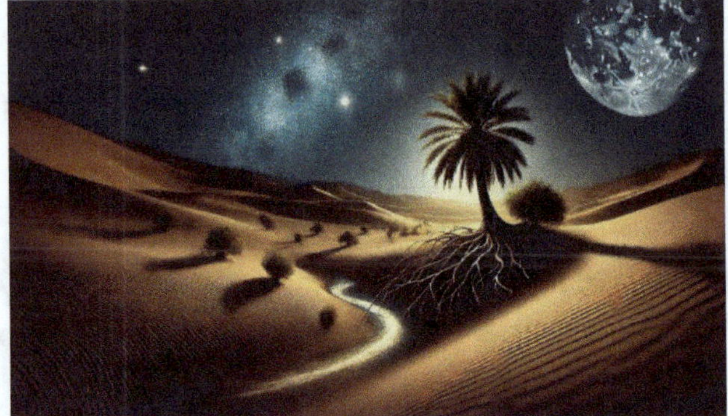 it stopped and took root definitively, giving life to the first palm grove. This fantastic story reflects the vital importance of palm trees in arid deserts and their spiritual connection to water, a symbol of life.

The palm trees that greet the Prophet

A traditional Islamic tale tells that when the Prophet Muhammad (peace be upon him) entered Medina during Hijra (emigration from Mecca to Medina), date palms tilted towards him as a sign of respect and blessing. Although this episode is not confirmed in major canonical texts such as the Qur'an or authentic hadiths, it is rich in symbolism and deeply rooted in the Islamic popular imagination, reflecting love and veneration for the Prophet. Muhammad's arrival in Medina marked the beginning of a new era for Islam, with the foundation of a community based on the values of justice, brotherhood and faith. The story of the palm trees bowing symbolizes the blessing of this city and the welcome that the inhabitants reserved for the Prophet. The act of palm trees could be seen as a reflection of the joy and universal respect for its arrival. In addition to the spiritual dimension, the story of the palms bending before the Prophet conveys a message of humility and veneration. The trees, rooted in the earth and reaching towards the sky, represent the balance between the earthly and spiritual worlds. Their inclination towards Muhammad underscores the recognition of his mission as a divine guide and messenger.

The crying palm tree

One of the most poignant authentic hadiths in Islamic tradition relates that a palm tree trunk uttered a desperate lament when the Prophet Muhammad (peace be upon him) stopped preaching near it and moved to a new minbar (pulpit).

According to the hadith, the Prophet Muhammad used to preach leaning against a palm trunk in the mosque of Medina. When a new minbar was built to facilitate preaching, he began to use it. At that moment, the trunk let out an audible wail, like that of a crying child. The Prophet, noticing the crying, approached the trunk and hugged it, consoling it until it calmed down. Then he told those present that the trunk was weeping because it no longer heard the recitation of the Word of Allah.

This episode, recorded in collections such as Sahih al-Bukhari and Sahih Muslim, is a manifestation of the unique character of the prophetic mission. It is not just a supernatural event, but a message for humanity. It shows that the whole of creation is interconnected and that the Prophet Muhammad was truly a universal figure, loved not only by men, but also by nature.

Symbolic Meaning in the Qur'an

The palm tree as a metaphor for faith

In the Quran, the palm tree is often associated with firmness and spiritual strength. Just as the roots of the palm tree penetrate deeply into the ground, the faithful must firmly root their faith. The crown of the palm tree, which rises towards the sky, represents the soul's aspiration towards God.

Date bunches as a reward sign

Sweet and nutritious dates are seen as a tangible sign of the rewards that await believers both in this life and in the afterlife. The role of dates in the Qur'an and in Islamic tradition goes far beyond their food value. They are a symbol of divine grace, a means of spiritual reflection and a deep connection between humanity and nature. Fantastic stories related to palm trees enrich this narrative, making dates a living metaphor for life, faith, and hope.

Chapter 5: Nutritional Properties of Dates

Dates are one of the most complete and nutritious food sources, combining natural sweetness, energy, and a wide range of essential nutrients. This chapter explores in detail the nutritional profile of dates and their culinary use, with a focus on traditional and modern recipes.

Nutritional Composition of Dates

Energy and Natural Sugars

Dates are rich in natural sugars such as glucose, fructose, and sucrose, making them an immediate source of energy.

They are especially popular with athletes and during Ramadan to break the fast, providing a quick calorie intake without overloading the digestive system.

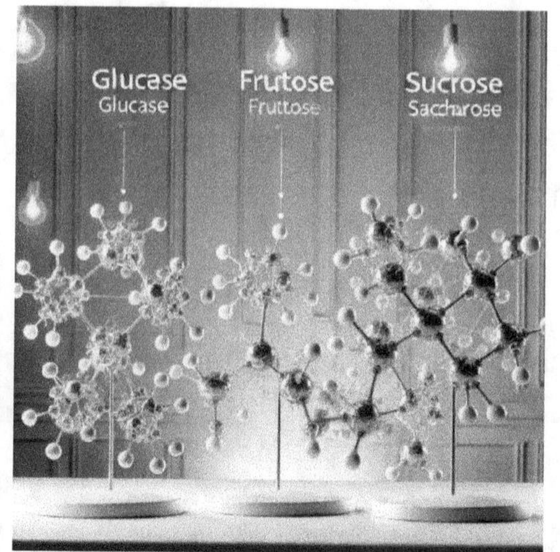

Calories: 20-25 kcal per date (on average 7-8 grams).
Sugars: Approximately 70-80% of the total weight, varying between varieties (e.g., Medjool dates are higher in sugar than Deglet Noor).

Dietary Fiber

Dates contain about 6-8 grams of fibres per 100 grams, contributing to digestive health. Soluble fibres promote cholesterol control, while insoluble fibres help intestinal transit.

Essential Minerals

- **Potassium:** Essential for muscle function and blood pressure regulation. Dates contain about 650 mg of potassium per 100 grams.
- **Magnesium:** Important for bone health and energy metabolism.
- **Calcium and Phosphorus:** Support bone and dental health.
- **Iron:** Beneficial for the prevention of anaemia, especially useful for women and during pregnancy.

Vitamin

- **Vitamin B6 (Pyridoxine):** Promotes the production of serotonin and norepinephrine, improving mood.
- **Vitamin A:** Present in small amounts, it is beneficial for eye and skin health.
- **Vitamin K:** Supports blood clotting and bone health.

Protein: About 2% of the total weight, with a balanced amino acid composition.

Dates contain small but significant amounts of amino acids, including:

- **Leucine and Isoleucine:** Important for muscle regeneration.
- **Lysine:** Essential for protein synthesis and strengthening the immune system.

Fats

Dates contain a very low amount of fat (0.1-0.4%), but those present are healthy fats. Here are the main types of fats found in dates:

- **Saturated fatty acids**: Palmitic: It is one of the saturated fatty acids found in dates, although in limited quantities.
- **Monounsaturated fatty acids**: Oleic: This monounsaturated fatty acid is beneficial for cardiovascular health and is present in small amounts in dates.
- **Polyunsaturated fatty acids**: Linoleic (omega-6): It is an essential fatty acid that the body cannot produce on its own. Supports skin and cell health. Linolenic (omega-3): May be present in trace amounts and has anti-inflammatory properties.

Nutritional Benefits

- **Immediate source of energy:** Thanks to simple carbohydrates, dates are ideal for recharging energy quickly.
- **Digestive support:** Fibres help prevent constipation and improves the health of the gut microbiota.
- **Cholesterol control:** Dates are cholesterol-free and can help lower LDL cholesterol levels.
- **Cardiovascular well-being:** The potassium and magnesium content supports heart health and blood pressure regulation.

Date Varieties and Nutritional Differences

Each variety of date has a unique nutritional profile:
- **Medjool:** Soft, large and high in sugar (often considered the "kings of dates").

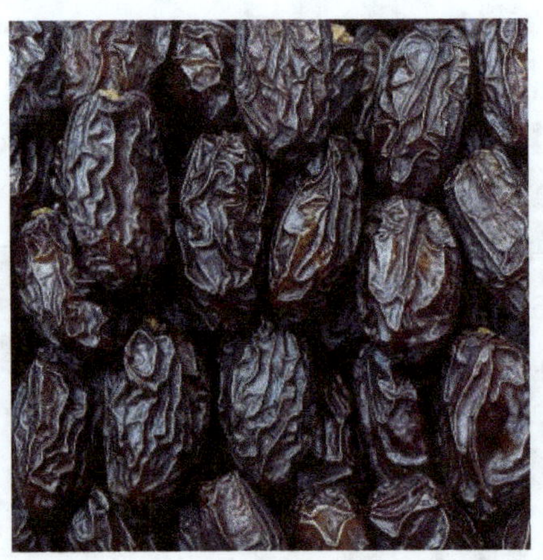

- **Deglet Noor:** Smaller and less sweet, ideal for baking.

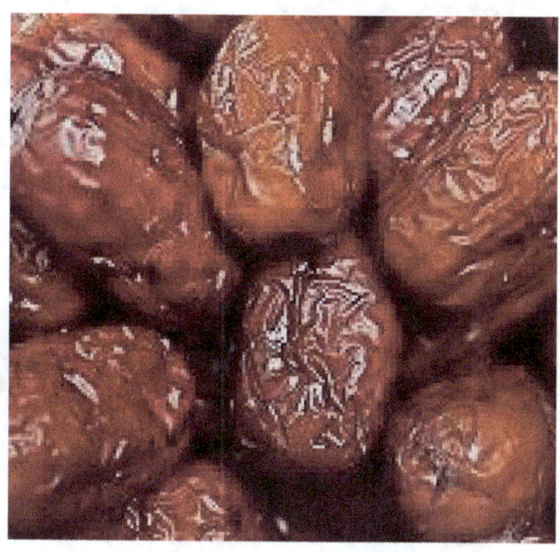

- **Ajwa:** Traditional Saudi Arabian foods, famous for their medicinal benefits.

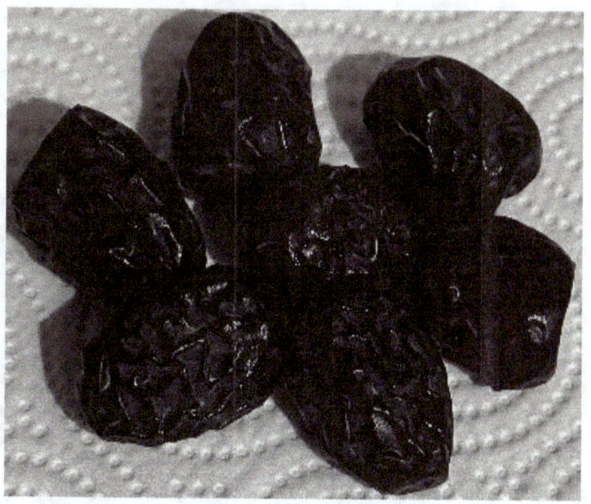

- **Sukkari:** delicious Arabian dates with a hint of honey and marron glacé

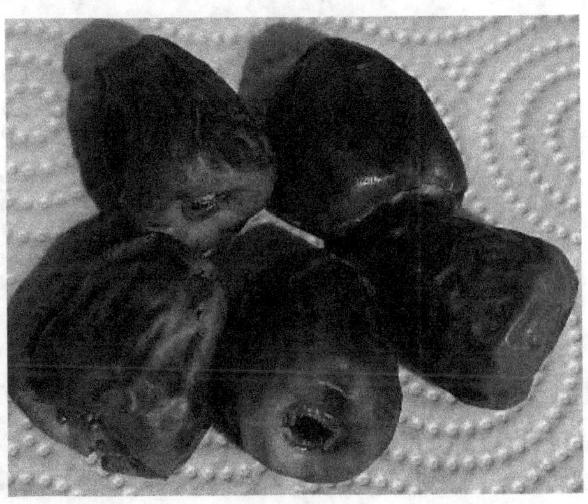

- **Khudri:** delicious Arabian dates with notes of raisins and honey

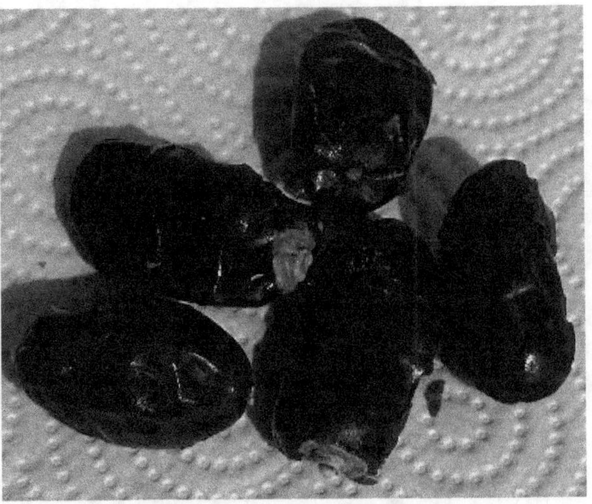

-   **Barhi:** Sweet and soft, often eaten fresh.

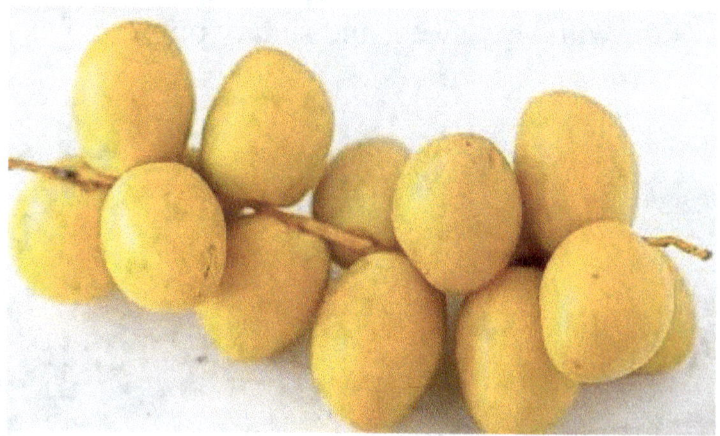

-   **Zahdi:** its origin dates to ancient Mesopotamia. It produces medium-sized, cylindrical fruits of a beautiful golden-brown colour that are sold semi-dry.

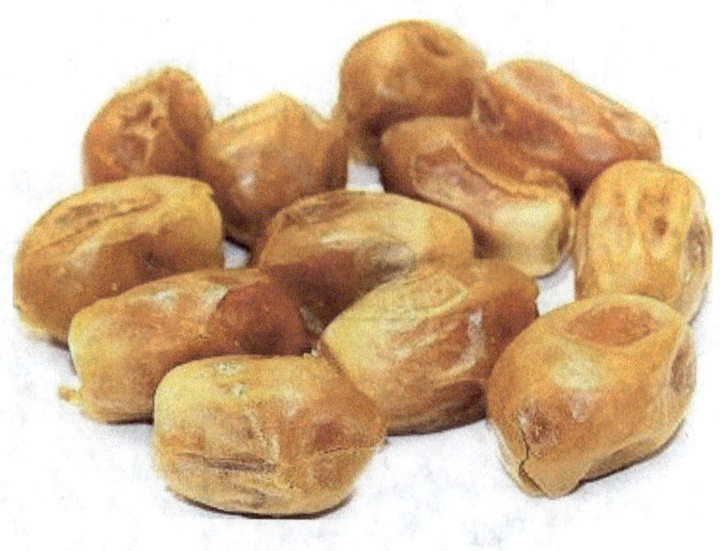

- **Sayer:** the fresh fruits are massively exported to Europe. The fruits are brown with orange hues, medium-sized, soft, with very sweet and sugary pulp.

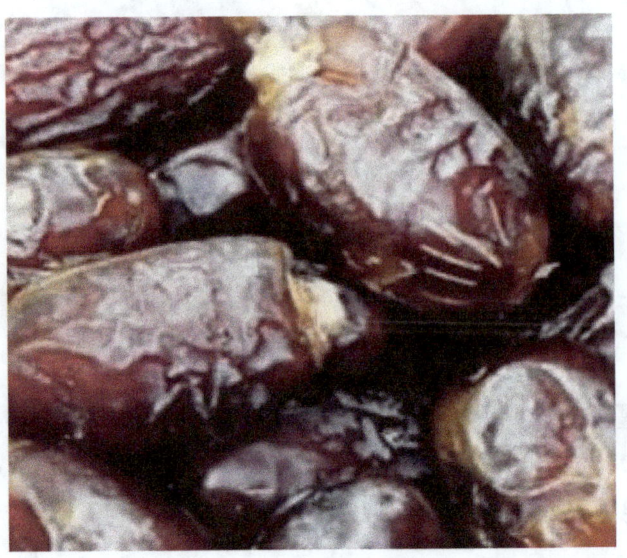

- **Khadrawy** produces dates that are marketed fresh and are particularly popular with Arabs.

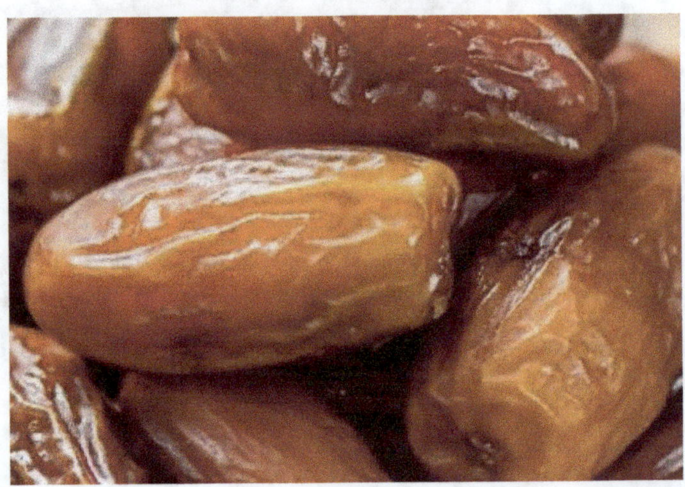

Dates in the Kitchen: Traditional and Modern Recipes

Dates are extremely versatile and lend themselves to a variety of culinary uses, from sweet to savory dishes

Sweet Recipes

Date brownies (sugar-free)

Ingredients: Medjool dates, cocoa powder, almonds, coconut oil.
Method: Blend the dates with almonds and cocoa. Roll out the dough and cool in the refrigerator. Cut into squares and serve.
Benefit: A healthy dessert, free of refined sugars.

Date Halwa

Tradition: Middle Eastern dessert made with dates, clarified butter and cardamom.
Method: Cook the dates with ghee and cardamom, adding toasted walnuts.

Dates Energy Balls

Ingredients: Dates, oats, walnuts, Chia seeds.
Method: Mix the ingredients in a blender, form balls and store in the refrigerator.

Savoury recipes

Dates stuffed with cheese

Ingredients: Deglet Noor dates, cream or goat cheese, walnuts.
Method: Remove the pit, fill with cheese and garnish with walnuts.
Benefit: Ideal as an elegant appetizer.

Salad with Dates and Oranges

Ingredients: Arugula, sliced dates, oranges, almonds, honey vinaigrette.
Method: Mix the ingredients and season with the vinaigrette.

Lamb tagine with dates

Tradition: Moroccan dish in which dates are cooked with meat, spices (turmeric, cinnamon) and almonds.
Method: Slowly cook the lamb with onions, spices and dates, serving with couscous.

Drinks and Snacks

Date Milk

Method: Blend dates with hot milk and a pinch of cinnamon. Ideal for an energetic breakfast.

Date and Banana Smoothie

Ingredients: Dates, bananas, almond milk.
Benefit: Rich in potassium and ideal for athletes.

Date Bars

Ingredients: Dates, sunflower seeds, almonds, honey.
Method: Mix and press into a baking dish, cool and cut.

Dates are an extraordinarily complete food, able to satisfy not only nutritional but also culinary needs, thanks to their versatility. Their natural sweetness, combined with their rich nutrient profile, makes them a valuable ingredient in both traditional and modern recipes. Rediscovering dates means approaching a healthy, balanced and respectful way of eating.

Chapter 6: Biochemical Properties of Dates

Dates are not only a source of energy and nutrition, but they contain a complex biochemical profile that makes them a functional food with numerous natural medicinal properties. This chapter explores the chemical composition of dates, their applications in pharmacology, and their uses in traditional and ancient medicine.

Chemical Composition of Dates

Dates contain a wide range of bioactive compounds responsible for their pharmacological benefits. Among the main ones:

- **Polyphenols:** Bioactive compounds that act as powerful antioxidants. Phenolic acids such as gallic, caffeic and ferulic acid are present in dates.
- **Flavonoids:** Compounds with anti-inflammatory, antimicrobial, and anticarcinogenic properties.
- **Phytosterols:** Reduction of LDL cholesterol and improvement of cardiovascular health.
- **Natural Sugars**: Glucose, fructose and sucrose, which provide immediate energy without the negative effect of refined sugars.
- **Minerals and Trace Elements**: Magnesium, iron, potassium and zinc, essential for enzymatic functions and metabolism.
- **Amino acids**: Including lysine, arginine and glycine, which contribute to overall well-being and support cell regeneration.
- **Alkaloids and Saponins**: Compounds found in small amounts that possess antimicrobial and anti-inflammatory activities.

The nutritional composition of date varieties is different especially for carbohydrates, proteins, dietary fibres, minerals and vitamins and is influenced by the stage of ripeness and drying:

- **Carbohydrates**: 44–88% (total sugars).
- **Fat**: 0.2–0.5%.
- **Proteins**: 2.3–5.6%.
- **Dietary fibres**: 6.4–11.5%.
- **Minerals**: Up to 916 mg/100 g dried dates.
- **Vitamins**: Vitamin C, B1, B2, A, riboflavin, niacin.

While it remains stable for antioxidant properties:

- **TPC** (total phenolic content): 172–246 mg GAE/100 g.
- **AA** (antioxidant activity): 146–162 μmol Vitamin E equivalents per gram.

Consuming them fresh or dried affects the antioxidant content, <u>with fresh dates generally richer in vitamin C, while dried ones maintain more stable levels of polyphenols and carotenoids.</u>
The focus on natural antioxidants, particularly those found in fruits, has grown due to their potential to fight free radicals and promote health. These compounds could represent an important resource in the prevention of chronic diseases related to oxidative stress.

Pharmacological properties

The unique combination of chemical compounds in dates has been shown to have multiple beneficial health effects.

Antibacterial and Antiviral

The bioactive compounds of dates, among which tannins stand out, have scientific evidence of antibacterial activity. Tannins are a class of polyphenolic compounds found in many plants, fruits, seeds, and bark. Their biological activity has been extensively studied, with particular attention to their antibacterial properties. These compounds act on different cellular mechanisms of bacteria, making them potential natural antimicrobial agents useful in healthcare, food and veterinary settings.

Mechanisms of action:

- Damage to the Cell Membrane: tannins can interact with proteins and lipids in the bacterial cell membrane, causing them to disintegrate and increasing permeability. This leads to the loss of essential ions and metabolites and the death of the bacterial cell.
- Enzymatic Inhibition: tannins bind to essential bacterial enzymes, inhibiting key reactions for the survival of the microorganism. Enzymes involved in protein synthesis and DNA replication are particularly sensitive.
- Chelation of Essential Metals: The ability of tannins to chelate metal ions, such as iron, prevents bacteria from using them for critical metabolic processes.
- Inhibition of Cell Wall Synthesis: Some studies suggest that tannins interfere with the synthesis of

peptidoglycan, an essential component of the cell wall in Gram-positive bacteria.
- Formation of Protein Complexes: Tannins form strong bonds with proteins, preventing them from functioning properly. This can affect bacterial adhesion and biofilm formation.

Tannins show activity against a broad spectrum of bacteria, both Gram-positive and Gram-negative. Some examples include:
- Gram-positive bacteria: Staphylococcus aureus, Streptococcus spp., Enterococcus spp.
- Gram-negative bacteri: Escherichia coli, Pseudomonas aeruginosa, Salmonella spp.

1. Food Industry: Tannins are used as natural preservatives to prevent microbial growth in food.
2. Medicine and Pharmaceuticals: they can be used as natural antimicrobial agents for the treatment of antibiotic-resistant bacterial infections.
3. Veterinary: Supplements containing tannins are used to improve intestinal health and prevent infections in ruminants and other animals.
4. Cosmetics: Tannins are included in skincare formulations due to their antimicrobial and antioxidant properties.

Despite their promising antibacterial properties, tannins have some limitations:

1. Chemical Stability: They can degrade easily under certain environmental conditions.
2. Toxicity: In very high doses (not present in fruits, but only possibly in concentrated extracts), they can also be toxic to host cells.
3. Microbial resistance: as with all drugs with antibacterial activity, it is possible that bacterial forms are also resistant to tannins.

Use of Dates in Traditional Medicine

Dates have been used for centuries as a natural remedy in different medical traditions, from Ayurveda to Arabic medicine.

Arabic and Islamic Medicine

1. **Energy and vitality:** Dates were consumed to provide immediate energy to desert travellers.
2. **Treatment of constipation:** The fibre found in dates were used to improve bowel function.
3. **Childbirth support:** Women consumed dates to facilitate labour, as suggested in the Quran (Surah of Mary).
4. **Action against poisons:** Hadith narrate that seven Ajwa dates a day protect against toxins and magic.

Ayurvedic Medicine

- **Body strengthening:** Dates, called *khajoor*, were used to increase physical strength and improve male fertility.
- **Remedies for the respiratory system:** Date decoctions were given to soothe coughs and relieve cold symptoms.

Traditional Chinese Medicine

- **Tone of yin:** Dates were considered a warming food, useful for rebalancing vital energy.
- **Anaemia:** They were used to treat weakness and anaemia, due to their high iron content.

Traditional Medicinal Prescriptions with Dates

Date decoction for the Respiratory System

- **Ingredients:** 5 dates, 2 cups of water, fresh ginger.
- **Procedure:** Boil the dates with ginger for 15 minutes. Strain and drink hot.
- **Benefit:** Soothes coughs and relieves congestion.

Date Paste for Energy and Fertility

- **Ingredients:** Dates, ghee, almonds, cardamom powder.
- **Procedure:** Blend the dates with hot ghee, add almonds and cardamom.
- **Benefit:** Strengthens the reproductive system and increases energy.

Date Milk for Postpartum Recovery

- **Ingredients:** 7 dates, 1 glass of hot milk.
- **Procedure:** Blend dates with milk and drink in the morning.
- **Benefit:** Promotes postpartum recovery and supports breast milk production.

Dates Soaked in Vinegar for Cholesterol

- **Ingredients:** Dried dates, apple cider vinegar.
- **Procedure:** Soak the dates in vinegar overnight and consume 1-2 in the morning.
- **Benefit:** Helps lower LDL cholesterol.

Modern Innovations and Applications in Pharmacology

Thanks to their chemical properties, dates are the subject of research for the development of new products:

Food Supplements
Date extracts are used to create antioxidant supplements and natural tonics.

Cosmetics
The phenolic compounds in dates are used in anti-aging creams and skin products.

Natural Medicines
Date extracts are studied for the treatment of diabetes, bacterial infections and neurodegenerative diseases.
The unique combination of chemical and pharmacological properties makes dates an extraordinary medicine-food, appreciated both in ancient traditions and in modern science.

Rediscovering their use in traditional medicine, integrating it with today's knowledge, offers new perspectives for health and well-being.

Chapter 7: Antioxidant and Anti-Inflammatory Properties of Dates

Antioxidants and Free Radicals

What are reactive free radicals?
Free radicals are highly reactive molecules that are naturally formed in our body during life processes. Despite their bad reputation, they are an essential part of our biology and play an ambivalent role: they can be both beneficial and harmful depending on the context and balance in our body. They are molecules or atoms that have an unpaired electron. This makes them unstable and very reactive, as they tend to "steal" an electron from other molecules to stabilize themselves. This process is called oxidation. Free radicals are formed as a byproduct of many normal and natural processes in our body, such as:

- Cellular respiration: During energy production in cells, a small amount of oxygen is transformed into free radicals.
- Immune system activity: When the body fights infection, it produces free radicals to destroy bacteria and viruses.
- Exposure to external factors: Radiation, pollution, cigarette smoke, alcohol, excess exercise, and certain chemicals can increase the production of free radicals.

Despite their reputation as "harmful molecules", free radicals perform some fundamental functions for our body:
- Fighting infections: Free radicals produced by the immune system destroy pathogenic microorganisms.
- Cell signaling: They help regulate cellular processes and communicate between cells.
- Adaptation to exercise: They stimulate the strengthening of the body's antioxidant defenses during physical activity.

They are molecules such as:
- the superoxide anion (O_2-) which contains both a negative electric charge and an unpaired electron and is therefore an anion and a radical at the same time (radical ion).
- the hydroxyl radical (-OH) is one of the reactive oxygen species (ROS); it is a molecule very important for cellular health and physiology because, in biological systems, it can radicalize numerous classes of molecules, including lipids. In cells, for example, it is responsible for the so-called lipid peroxidation involving the lipids of the cell membrane.
- the peroxyl radical (RO•).

If not managed properly, free radicals can cause significant damage to the body. The chemical reactions they trigger can damage crucial molecules such as lipids, proteins, and nucleic acids (DNA), contributing to aging processes and chronic diseases.
- DNA damage: Free radicals can damage DNA, causing genetic mutations that can lead to diseases such as cancer in the long run. This damage can interfere with proper DNA replication, leading to cellular errors that can result in tumours.

- Cellular aging: Free radicals are closely linked to the aging process. The cellular damage caused by these molecules leads to a reduction in the efficiency of tissues and biological systems, causing greater vulnerability to disease.
- Cardiovascular disease: The oxidation of lipids (especially LDL cholesterol) by free radicals is a major cause of atherosclerosis, which can lead to cardiovascular diseases such as heart attack and stroke.
- Neurodegenerative diseases: Oxidative damage is also involved in neurodegenerative diseases such as Alzheimer's disease and Parkinson's, in which nerve cell damage impairs brain function.

What harmful effects do they have on the human body?
Free radicals can cause:
- Alteration of membrane fluidity.
- Protein denaturation.
- Lipid peroxidation.
- Oxidative damage to DNA.
- Alteration of platelet functions (Fridovich, 1978; Kinsella et al., 1993).

These effects are associated with chronic health problems, such as cancer, inflammation, aging, and atherosclerosis.

<u>Antioxidants are molecules that neutralize free radicals</u>, reducing or preventing oxidative damage to cells and tissues. Antioxidants may have positive effects in **the prevention of degenerative diseases** (Shahidi, 1997). Their ability to eliminate free radicals makes them relevant in reducing the risk of chronic diseases (Silva et al., 2007).

Phytocompounds derived from fruits show significant **antioxidant capacity**. These compounds are related to **lower incidence and mortality** from degenerative diseases in humans (Javanmardi et al., 2003).

Antioxidants can be of natural or synthetic origin. Both play an essential role in protecting against oxidative damage, but have differences in terms of chemical structure, efficacy and applications.

Natural antioxidants are compounds found in food, plants, and living organisms. They can be obtained through the diet and play a vital role in biological protection.

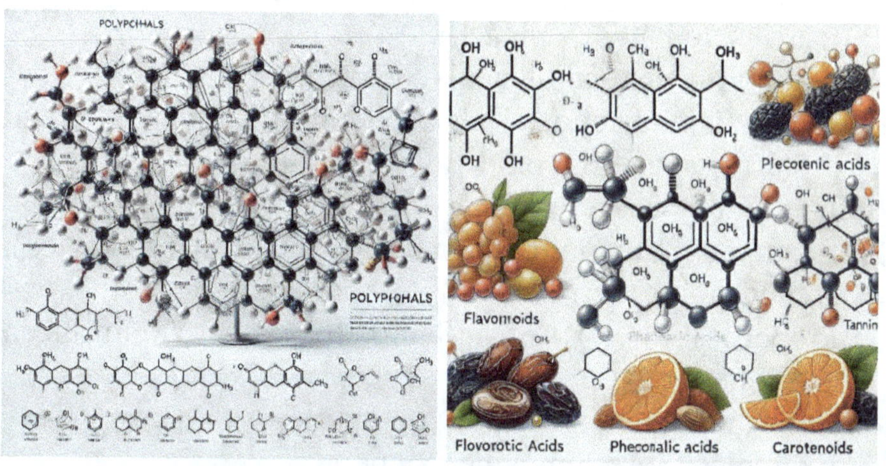

Main types of natural antioxidants:

Polyphenols
1. Sources: Fruits, vegetables, green tea, cocoa, red wine.
2. Examples: Flavonoids, gallic acid, resveratrol.

3. Mechanism of action: They reduce ROS due to their ability to donate electrons or hydrogens, stabilizing free radicals.

Antioxidant vitamins

1. Vitamin C (ascorbic acid): Present in citrus fruits, kiwis, peppers.
2. Vitamin E (tocopherols and tocotrienols): It is found in vegetable oils, nuts and seeds.
3. Mechanism of action: They inhibit the oxidation of lipids in cell membranes and protect tissues from oxidative damage.

Carotenoids

1. Sources: Orange, red and green fruits and vegetables (carrots, tomatoes, spinach).
2. Examples: Beta-carotene, lycopene, lutein.
3. Mechanism of action: They absorb the energy of ROS and protect tissues from oxidation.

Specific phenolic compounds

1. Examples: Curcumin (turmeric), catechins (green tea), anthocyanins (berries).
2. Properties: Anti-inflammatory, anticancer, cardioprotective.

Antioxidant minerals

1. Examples: Selenium, zinc, copper.
2. Role: Cofactors for antioxidant enzymes such as glutathione peroxidase and superoxide dismutase.

What advantages natural antioxidants offer:
- **Biocompatibility:** They are easily metabolized by the body.

- **Multifunctional activity:** They often combine antioxidant properties with anti-inflammatory and anticancer activities.
- **Presence in balanced diets:** They contribute to the prevention of chronic diseases such as diabetes, cardiovascular disease and cancer.

Among the disadvantages we have:
- **Chemical stability:** Some natural antioxidants, such as vitamin C, are sensitive to heat, light, and oxygen.
- **Variable bioavailability:** Not all natural antioxidants are easily absorbed or used by the body.

Synthetic antioxidants are chemically produced molecules, mainly used to preserve food, pharmaceuticals and cosmetic products. They are designed to mimic or amplify the action of natural antioxidants.

The main synthetic antioxidants are:
1. <u>Butylhydroxytoluene (BHT) and Butylated hydroxyanisole (BHA)</u>
   - Applications: Preservative function in packaged foods, cosmetics and industrial products.
   - Mechanism of action: They inhibit lipid oxidation in products, increasing shelf life.
2. <u>Tert- butylhydroquinone (TBHQ)</u>
   - Use: Storage of edible oils and fats.
   - Features: High chemical stability and efficacy at low concentrations.
3. <u>Propyl gallate</u>
   - Application: Protection of fatty foods against rancidity.
   - Mechanism of action: Donate electrons to free radicals, disrupting oxidative chain reactions.

What benefits do synthetic antioxidants offer?

1. **Lower Cost:** They are cheap to produce on a large scale.
2. **High stability:** They are more resistant to degradation than many natural antioxidants.
3. **Specificity:** They can be formulated to act on certain types of free radicals or environmental conditions.

However, beware of the disadvantages among which the following are reported in the bibliography:

1. **Potential negative health effects:** Some synthetic antioxidants, such as BHT and BHA, have been associated with long-term adverse effects, including possible carcinogenicity in high doses.
2. **Consumer acceptance:** The preference for "natural" ingredients has reduced the popularity of synthetic antioxidants in many industries.

Characteristics between natural and synthetic antioxidants table 1:

Characteristic	Natural Antioxidants	Synthetic Antioxidants
Source	Food, plants, living organisms	Chemical synthesis
Effectiveness	Bioavailability dependent	High stability and specificity
Safety	Generally safe	Potential side effects
Stability	Sensitive to heat and light	Very stable
Cost	Can be elevated	Cost-effective on a large scale

Dates are a rich source of antioxidants, the type and quantity of which can vary significantly between different varieties. Antioxidants found in dates include polyphenolic compounds, carotenoids, and vitamin C, which help fight free radicals and improve overall health. Dates contain phenolic acids such as gallic, caffeic and ferulic acids.

Neuroprotective Activity of Polyphenols

Polyphenols are natural bioactive compounds found in a wide range of plant foods such as fruits, vegetables, tea, grapes, and cocoa. In recent years, numerous studies have highlighted their neuroprotective potential, making them the subject of great interest in the prevention and treatment of neurodegenerative diseases such as Alzheimer's, Parkinson's and other conditions related to brain aging.

- **Antioxidant Action**: Polyphenols neutralize free radicals and reduce oxidative stress, a key factor in the onset of neuronal damage.
- **Modulation of Inflammatory Pathways**: They intervene in the cell signalling pathways involved in inflammatory processes, reducing the production of pro-inflammatory cytokines.
- **Neuronal Cell Protection**: They promote neuronal survival through the activation of neurotrophic pathways, such as the brain-derived neurotrophic factor (BDNF) pathway.
- **Reduction of Toxic Protein Accumulation**: Certain polyphenols can prevent the aggregation of pathological proteins, such as beta-amyloid and alpha-synuclein, associated with neurodegenerative diseases.
- **Improved Mitochondrial Function**: They improve cellular bioenergetics and reduce mitochondrial dysfunction, a crucial aspect in neurodegeneration.

<u>Types of antioxidants found in dates:</u>

1. **Polyphenols**
   - Main compounds: Flavonoids, phenolic acids and tannins.
   - Effects: Reduction of oxidative stress, anti-inflammatory properties and anti-carcinogenic potential.
2. **Carotenoids**
   - Main compounds: Lutein and beta-carotene.
   - Effects: Protecting cells from damage caused by free radicals and improving vision health.

3. **Vitamin C**
   - Mainly found in fresh dates.
   - Effects: Strengthens the immune system and contributes to the neutralization of free radicals.

Comparison of date varieties table 2

Variety	Polyphenols	Carotenoids	Vitamin C	Main features
Medjool	Very high	Moderate	Low (dried)	Rich in flavonoids and tannins, ideal for cardiovascular protection.
Deglet Nour	Moderate	Moderate	Low	They contain balanced levels of antioxidants, which are beneficial for overall health.
Barhi	Elevated (fresh)	High	Treble (fresh)	Particularly rich in carotenoids and vitamin C in the fresh phase.
Zahidi	Moderate	Low	Low	Less rich in antioxidants than other varieties, but with a stable profile.
Ajwa	Very high	Moderate	Low	Exceptionally rich in flavonoids and polyphenols, known for anti-inflammatory properties.

Summary of the differences in antioxidants of date varieties:

- **Medjool dates**: Among the richest in polyphenols, they are ideal for those looking for long-term antioxidant benefits, especially for cardiovascular health.
- **Deglet Nour Dates**: They offer a balanced profile, suitable for daily use and general support against oxidative stress.
- **Barhi dates**: Excellent source of antioxidants in their fresh phase due to the high content of vitamin C and carotenoids. Their antioxidant power decreases with drying.
- **Zahidi dates**: They contain lower amounts of antioxidants, but they are still helpful in maintaining a healthy diet.
- **Ajwa Dates**: Known to be one of the richest varieties in antioxidants, they are often considered a functional food due to their therapeutic properties.

The choice of date variety depends on your specific needs:

- For **high antioxidant benefits**, **Medjool** and **Ajwa** varieties are best.
- For a higher content of **vitamin C** and **carotenoids**, **fresh Barhi dates** are preferable.
- For a **balanced profile and culinary versatility**, **Deglet Nours** are a good option.

Anti-Inflammatory Properties of Dates

Chronic inflammation is the basis of many degenerative diseases. Dates are rich in bioactive compounds that help regulate the inflammatory response.

Anti-inflammatory activities

Polyphenols and other natural antioxidants show significant anti-inflammatory properties, acting primarily through modulation of inflammatory cytokines. Their ability to regulate inflammatory processes is crucial for the treatment of chronic diseases such as rheumatoid arthritis, cardiovascular disease and neurodegenerative conditions.

Mechanisms of action

1. **Reduction of Pro-inflammatory Cytokines:** Pro-inflammatory cytokines are proteins produced by the immune system that play a crucial role in activating and regulating the inflammatory response. Although inflammation is a natural defensive response of the body to infection or tissue damage, chronic overactivation of pro-inflammatory cytokines has been associated with numerous diseases, including arthritis, cardiovascular disease, diabetes, and neurodegenerative diseases. Polyphenols can adjust cytokine production and activity due to their antioxidant properties. They act through several mechanisms, including:
   - Inhibition of inflammatory pathways: Polyphenols may reduce the activation of certain cellular pathways that promote inflammation, such as the NF-kB and MAPK pathway, a key pathway in the regulation of pro-inflammatory cytokines.

- Reduction of oxidative stress: Since oxidative stress is a powerful trigger to produce inflammatory cytokines, polyphenols, by reducing free radicals, help prevent chronic inflammation.
- Modulation of immune cells: Polyphenols can directly affect the activity of immune system cells, such as macrophages, which are involved in the production of inflammatory cytokines. In this way, polyphenols help balance the immune response, reducing inflammation.

2. **Inhibition of COX-2** (cicloossigenasi-2) **and iNOS** (Nitric oxide inductable synthase) **Expression**: These enzymes are involved in the synthesis of inflammatory mediators such as prostaglandins and nitric oxide. Polyphenols reduce its activity.

3. **Activation of Antioxidant Pathways**: Antioxidants activate enzymes such as superoxide dismutase (SOD) and catalase, reducing oxidative stress and subsequent inflammation. SOD is an enzyme that plays a very important role in our body, helping to protect cells from damage caused by free radicals. SOD can neutralize one of these free radicals called superoxide, which is a type of reactive oxygen. In practice, superoxide dismutase acts as a "scavenger" that sweeps away the superoxide, transforming it into other less harmful molecules, such as hydrogen peroxide (hydrogen peroxide), which in turn is transformed into water and oxygen by another enzyme. In this way, SOD helps maintain balance and protect cells from damage that could cause disease or premature aging.

4. **Immune Cell Modulation**: They affect the activity of macrophages, T lymphocytes, and other immune cells, promoting an anti-inflammatory response.
5. **Regulation of MicroRNAs (miRNAs):** Polyphenols can modulate the expression of specific miRNAs involved in the regulation of inflammatory cytokines. MicroRNAs (miRNAs) are small RNA molecules that do not code for proteins but play a critical role in regulating gene expression. In other words, miRNAs control which genes are turned on or off inside cells. These RNA molecules are about 22 nucleotides long and, by binding to specific messenger RNA (mRNA) sequences, prevent these mRNAs from being translated into proteins or degrade them. In the context of inflammation, miRNAs are involved in a variety of ways, as they can regulate the activity of numerous genes that participate in the inflammatory response. MiRNAs influence several cellular and molecular processes related to inflammation, such as the production of cytokines (the proteins that mediate inflammation), the immune response, and the migration of inflammatory cells to sites of damage.

Liver protection

Dates also protect the liver from damage caused by toxins thanks to their antioxidant activity. Studies in animal models have shown a significant reduction in liver damage after administration of date extracts. Chronic inflammation is one of the main contributing factors to liver damage and diseases such as fatty liver disease or cirrhosis. Flavonoids help reduce inflammation in the liver and improve liver health. The liver has a remarkable ability to regenerate, but in the event of severe damage, this ability can be impaired. Dates contain vitamins and minerals, such as potassium and magnesium, which support cellular metabolism and can stimulate liver cell regeneration and repair.

Examples of Polyphenols with Anti-Inflammatory Properties

- Curcumin: Suppresses NF-κB activity and reduces levels of TNF-α (tumour necrosis factor) and IL-6.
- Quercetin: Inhibits COX-2 activity and regulates the production of pro-inflammatory cytokines. Reduces the production of **TNF-α** (tumour necrosis factor). In dates it is found in good quantities.
- Resveratrol: Modulates the activity of MAPK pathways and reduces oxidative stress.
- Epigallocatechin Gallate (EGCG): Potent inhibitor of IL-1β and TNF-α production.
- Phenolic Acids: They inhibit the production of pro-inflammatory molecules such as cytokines (e.g. IL-6, TNF-α) and enzymes involved in inflammatory processes (e.g. cyclooxygenase, COX-2, Lipoxygenase). There are good quantities in dates.

Scientific evidence

Date extracts have shown anti-inflammatory effects in models of arthritis and other inflammatory diseases. Studies in human cells indicate that the phenolic compounds in dates reduce oxidative stress in inflammatory cells.

Traditional Remedies of Indigenous and Rural Peoples

Date palms and their fruits have been used for centuries by indigenous and rural communities to treat inflammatory diseases and other ailments. Some significant examples:

Remedies for Gastrointestinal Inflammation

- **Populations of North Africa:** They prepared a decoction of dried dates to treat gastritis and ulcers. The fibre and polyphenol content helped reduce inflammation of the gastric mucosa.
- **Traditional remedy:** Date decoction with palm leaves is good to relieve heartburn.

Treatment of Respiratory Diseases

- **Arabian deserts:** For bronchitis and asthma, an infusion of fresh dates was prepared with ginger and honey, which soothed the respiratory tract and reduced inflammation.
- **Specific remedy:** Dates were roasted and crushed into powder, mixed with hot water to create a tonic for coughs and phlegm.

Topical Applications for Wounds and Skin Inflammation

- **Sub-Saharan Africa:** Date pulp mixed with honey and shea butter was applied to wounds to speed up healing.
- **South Asia:** Palm leaf and date extract was used to prepare compresses on inflamed or painful areas.

Arthritis and Muscle Pain

- **Traditional Arabic medicine:** Oil extracted from date seeds was massaged into sore joints to relieve symptoms of arthritis.
- **Date seed infusion:** An infusion of powdered seeds was drunk to reduce joint inflammation.

Antioxidant and Anti-Inflammatory Medicinal Prescriptions

Anti-inflammatory Herbal Tea with Dates

Ingredients: 5 dates, a teaspoon of turmeric, fresh ginger, a pinch of cinnamon.
Procedure: Boil dates with turmeric and ginger in 500 ml of water for 15 minutes. Strain and drink hot.
Benefits: Reduces inflammation and strengthens the immune system.

Date Wrap for Joint Pain

Ingredients: Date pulp, honey, olive oil.
Procedure: Crush the dates and mix with honey and oil. Apply the mixture to sore joints and wrap with a warm cloth.
Benefits: Reduces swelling and pain.

Antioxidant Energy Drink

Ingredients: 7 Medjool dates, almond milk, cocoa powder.
Procedure: Blend the dates with almond milk and add cocoa. Serve cold or hot.
Benefits: Provides energy and protects against chronic diseases.

Modern Innovations in the Use of Dates

The antioxidant and anti-inflammatory properties of dates are attracting the attention of scientific research and the pharmaceutical industry:

Pharmaceutical Extracts

Phenolic extracts from dates are used in dietary supplements for the prevention of chronic diseases.
Applications in natural medicines for the management of diabetes and inflammation.

Anti-Aging Cosmetics

Carotenoids and polyphenols from dates are included in creams to reduce signs of skin aging and protect against UV damage.

The antioxidant and anti-inflammatory properties of dates make them an irreplaceable food-medicine. From traditional indigenous remedies to modern applications, dates prove their value not only as a food, but also as a source of holistic well-being. Incorporating dates into your diet and inflammation treatment is a natural way to promote health and longevity.

Chapter 8: Sugars in Dates

Carbohydrates represent a class of macronutrients that are fundamental for human and animal nutrition, being one of the main sources of energy for the body. In addition to their energetic function, they play significant roles in overall health and well-being, thanks to their nutraceutical properties.

Classification and Sources

Carbohydrates can be divided into three main categories:

Simple sugars: monosaccharides (e.g. glucose, fructose) and disaccharides (e.g. sucrose, lactose). These are quickly digested and absorbed, providing immediate energy to the body.

Glucose ($C_6H_{12}O_6$): a monosaccharide essential for energy metabolism.

A 3D molecular representation of glucose. Show the cyclic form of glucose (pyranose structure) with carbon, hydrogen, and oxygen atoms labelled.

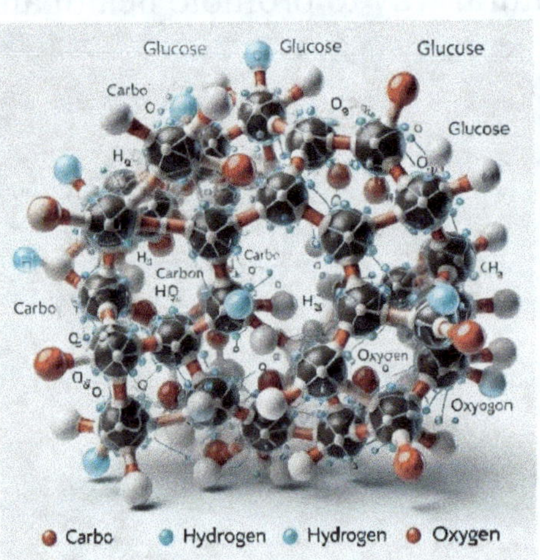

-   Fructose (C6H12O6): A monosaccharide found in fruit and honey.

Sucrose (C12H22O11): a disaccharide composed of glucose and fructose, found in fruits, honey, table sugar, milk.

A planar molecular representation of sucrose. Show the glucose and fructose units joined by an alpha-1,2-glycosidic bond.

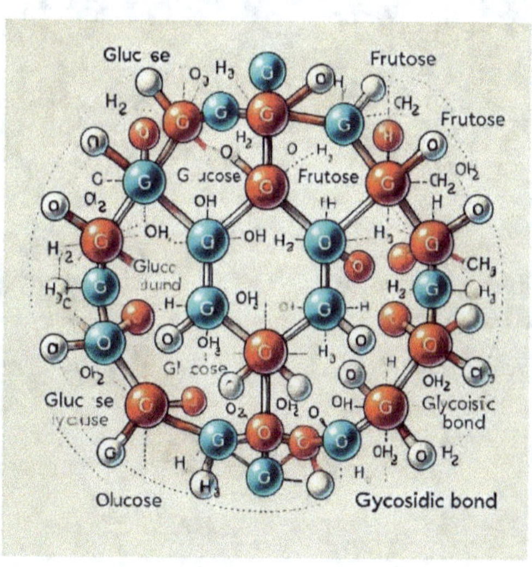

Complex carbohydrates: These include oligosaccharides and polysaccharides (e.g. starch and glycogen). These require longer digestion and release energy gradually.

Starches (($C6H10O5$)n): polysaccharide found in cereals and tubers.

A planar schematic representation of starch, combining amylose and amylopectin structures. Show linear chains of glucose units connected by alpha-1,4-glycosidic bonds for amylose, and branched chains with alpha-1,4 and alpha-1,6-glycosidic bonds for amylopectin.

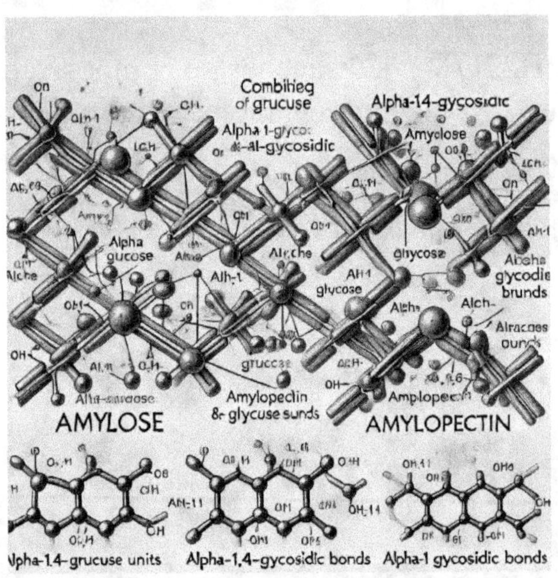

A planar schematic representation of amylopectin, showing its branched structure with glucose units connected by alpha-1,4-glycosidic bonds in the linear chains and alpha-1,6-glycosidic bonds at the branch points.

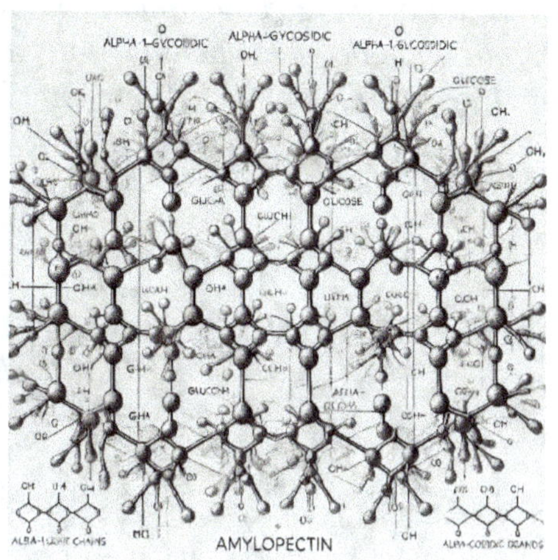

A 3D molecular representation of amylopectin, showcasing its complex branching structure. Highlight the glucose monomers interconnected by alpha-1,4-glycosidic bonds in the linear segments and alpha-1,6-glycosidic bonds at the branch points.

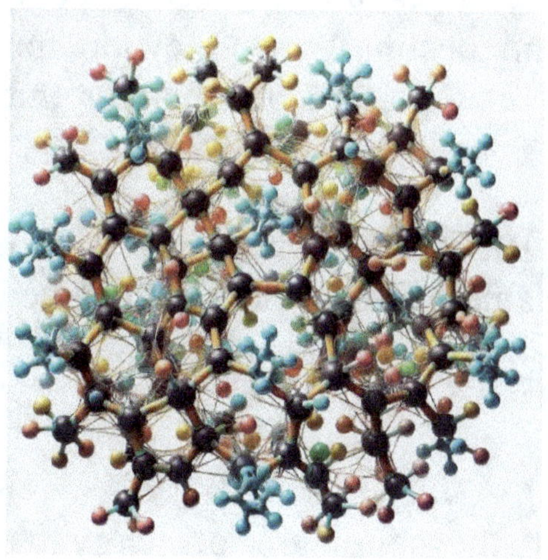

Glycogen ((C6H10O5)n): form of energy reserve in animals found in whole grains, legumes, tubers.

A schematic representation of the glycogen molecule in a planar formula style. The image should include a branching polymer of glucose units connected by alpha-1,4-glycosidic bonds in the main chain and alpha-1,6-glycosidic bonds at branch points.

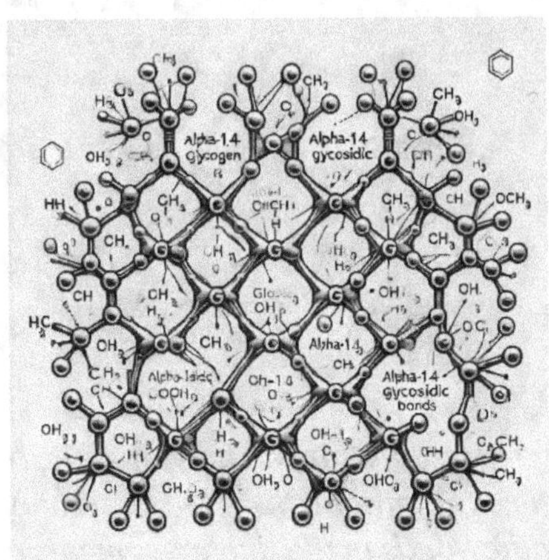

Dietary fibres: non-digestible polysaccharides such as cellulose, hemicellulose and pectin. While they do not provide direct energy, they have important benefits for gut and metabolic health.

Cellulose ((C6H10O5)n): structural polysaccharide of plants. It is found in vegetables, fruits, whole grains, seeds.

Nutritional effects

Energy Supply

Carbohydrates are the main source of energy for the human body, providing 4 kcal per gram. Glycolysis and the Krebs cycle convert glucose into ATP, the energy unit (fuel) used by cells.

Simple sugars provide immediate energy intake, while complex carbohydrates promote sustained release, keeping blood glucose levels stable.

Blood Sugar Control

Low glycaemic index (GI) carbohydrates help stabilize blood sugar levels, reducing the risk of hyperglycaemia and improving insulin sensitivity. These foods are especially beneficial for individuals with diabetes or metabolic syndrome.

Digestive Health

Insoluble fibres improve intestinal peristalsis, preventing constipation, while soluble fibres, such as pectin, form gels that promote the sense of satiety and regulate the absorption of fats and sugars.

Nutraceutical Effects

Prebiotics and Microbiota

Some carbohydrates, such as inulin and fructo-oligosaccharides (FOS), act as prebiotics, stimulating the growth of beneficial bacteria in the gut microbiota. A healthy microbiota is related to reduced inflammation and improved metabolism.

Cardiovascular Protection

Soluble fibres, such as that found in oats, can reduce LDL cholesterol levels, decreasing the risk of cardiovascular disease. In addition, foods rich in complex carbohydrates and fibres help keep blood pressure within healthy limits.

Antioxidant effects

Some carbohydrates, such as pectin and glucans, exhibit indirect antioxidant effects, promoting the reduction of oxidative stress in the body.

Recommended Consumption and Considerations

Nutritional guidelines suggest that carbohydrates should make up 45-65% of your daily calorie intake, favouring whole grain sources and limiting refined sugars to a maximum of 10% of total calories. Each gram of carbohydrate provides about 4 kcal. Excessive consumption of simple sugars is associated with obesity, dental caries, and increased risk of metabolic diseases. In contrast, the intake of complex carbohydrates and Fiber is related to numerous health benefits. Carbohydrates, if chosen wisely, can play a crucial role not only in meeting energy needs, but also in promoting general health and preventing various diseases. Supplementing with fibres-rich foods and low-GI carbohydrates is essential for a balanced and functional diet. At the same time, awareness of the risks associated with an excess of simple sugars is essential to minimize the negative effects of unbalanced consumption.

Sugars in Dates

Dates are naturally sweet, containing a combination of simple sugars that provide immediate energy.

Types of Sugars

1. **Glucose and Fructose:** Simple sugars that are quickly assimilated, present in high quantities.

2. **Sucrose:** Present in some varieties, less than glucose and fructose.
3. **Average Sugar Concentration:** Approximately 65-75% of the dry weight in dates, which varies depending on the variety. For example:
   - Medjool: High concentration of sugars (~75-80%).
   - Deglet Noor: Less concentration of sugars (~60-65%).

Glycaemic Index (GI) of Dates

The glycaemic index measures how quickly a food raises blood sugar levels.

Dates have a moderate GI (around 42-55), depending on the variety and degree of ripeness.

This makes them a more stable source of sugars than refined sweeteners but requires caution for diabetics.

Nutritional Recommendations

Alternative for Desserts

Dates can replace refined sugar in many recipes. For example:
Date puree: Blend dates with water to make a natural sweetener, useful for cakes or cookies.

Healthy Recipes with Dates

1. **Salad with Dates and Spinach**
   - Ingredients: Fresh spinach, sliced dates, walnuts, feta, olive oil.
   - Benefit: Rich in fibres and protein, with a low glycaemic impact.
2. **Date Energy Bars**
   - Ingredients: Dates, oatmeal, Chia seeds, almond butter.

- Indication: Excellent for sustained energy without glycaemic peaks.

The amino acids and sugars found in dates make them a nutritionally rich and beneficial food, but it is essential consume them consciously, especially for those with diabetes. When well-balanced in the diet, dates can offer valuable energy and nutrients without compromising glycaemic management. However, portion control and customizing consumption according to individual needs remain key to avoid risks.

Special attention for Diabetes

Type 1 diabetes

Type 1 diabetes is characterized by a total or partial lack of insulin. For insulin-dependent patients, the consumption of dates may be allowed by the doctor in limited amounts, but only if carefully balanced with the insulin administered. A possible indication could be to consume a few dates as a snack to prevent hypoglycaemia during physical activity. In all cases, excessive consumption should be avoided as it could cause a rapid glycaemic peak.

Type 2 diabetes

In type 2 diabetes, which is characterised by insulin resistance, date intake must be even more controlled. The indication could be to consume in moderation (1-2 dates per day) as part of a meal rich in fibres, protein and healthy fats, which reduce the overall glycaemic load. Even in this case, however, it is necessary to obtain medical advice.

In case of use, however, prefer varieties with a low sugar content, such as Deglet Noor and avoid Medjool dates or other very sugary varieties, especially if consumed alone.

Strategies for Consuming Dates Safely

1. **Combine them with Protein or Fiber:** Consume dates together with dried fruit (almonds, walnuts) or Greek yogurt to slow down the absorption of sugars.
2. **Portion control:** Limit consumption to 1-2 dates per serving.
3. **Monitor your blood sugar:** Check your blood sugar levels regularly to assess the impact of dates.

Benefits and Harms of Dates for Diabetics

Benefits:
1. Natural energy: Ideal for an immediate energy boost, such as before or after exercise.
2. Fiber: They promote digestion and help prevent sudden glycaemic spikes.
3. Minerals and antioxidants: They support cardiovascular health, which is often compromised in diabetics.

Risks:
1. Glycaemic load: High sugar content can cause blood sugar to rise rapidly when consumed in high amounts or without balance.
2. Calorie excess: Overweight diabetics must consider the calorie content of dates.

Chapter 9: Amino Acids in Dates

Amino acids are organic compounds that are critical to life, as they are the building blocks of proteins, essential for a wide range of biological functions. Every living organism is built and maintained thanks to these extraordinary molecules, which play vital roles in growth, tissue repair, and maintaining homeostasis.

Chemical Structure of Amino Acids

Chemically, amino acids consist of an amino group ($-NH_2$), a carboxyl group ($-COOH$), and a unique side chain (R) bonded to a central carbon (α-carbon). The variety and chemical characteristics of amino acids derive precisely from the different side chains.

The general structure is:

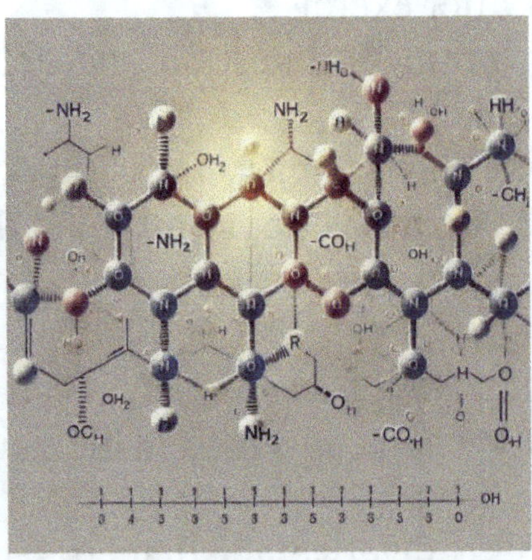

The (R) side chain determines the polarity, charge, and specific properties of the amino acid.

Classification of Amino Acids

Amino acids can be classified according to several criteria:
1. Essential amino acids: they cannot be synthesized by the body and must be obtained through the diet. They include leucine, isoleucine, lysine, methionine, phenylalanine, threonine, tryptophan and valine. In children, arginine is considered essential.
2. Non-essential amino acids: they can be synthesized by the body. They include alanine, asparagine, aspartic acid, glutamic acid, etc.

Chemical-physical properties

- Non-polar: Glycine, alanine, valine, leucine, isoleucine, methionine, proline.
- Uncharged polars: Serine, threonine, asparagine, glutamine.
- Acids: Aspartic acid, glutamic acid.
- Basics: Lysine, arginine, histidine.

Functions of Amino Acids

Amino acids perform numerous vital functions, including:
1. Protein synthesis: The main function of amino acids is to assemble into polypeptide chains, forming proteins that play structural, enzymatic and transport roles.
2. Energy production: Some amino acids can be used as an energy source through gluconeogenesis or ketogenesis.
3. Synthesis of biological molecules: They participate in the formation of hormones, neurotransmitters (such as dopamine and serotonin), and other essential molecules.

4. Detoxification and homeostasis: They contribute to balancing the body's pH and removing toxic waste products, such as ammonia.

Amino Acids and Nutrition

A balanced intake of amino acids is essential for maintaining good health. Dietary proteins are the main source of amino acids, and their quality depends on the content and proportion of essential amino acids.

Food Sources

- **Animals**: Meat, fish, eggs, dairy products (considered complete sources, as they contain all essential amino acids).
- **Vegetables:** Legumes, cereals, nuts and seeds (some may be deficient in one or more essential amino acids, for example lysine in cereals or methionine in legumes).

Protein Complementation

For vegetarians and vegans, combining different foods (such as grains and legumes) is essential to get all the amino acids you need.

Amino Acids and Health

A proper balance of amino acids is crucial for preventing deficiencies and metabolic disorders. Some examples:

1. Essential Amino Acid Deficiency: It can lead to problems such as growth retardation, loss of muscle mass, and weakened immune system.
2. Excess of certain amino acids: It can cause side effects such as liver or kidney toxicity (for example, from excessive consumption of protein supplements).

Branched Chain Amino Acids (BCAAs)

BCAAs (leucine, isoleucine and valine) are particularly important for athletes, because:
- They promote muscle protein synthesis.
- They help reduce catabolism during intense exercise.
- They improve muscle recovery.

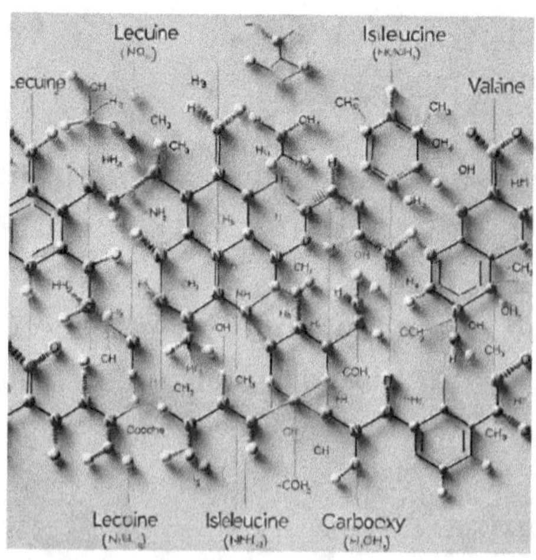

Amino acids are essential components for the proper functioning of our body. A varied and balanced diet is the best way to ensure an adequate intake of these valuable nutrients. Understanding their functions and role in health can help optimize overall well-being and prevent diseases related to nutritional imbalances.

Amino Acids in Dates

Amino acids are the building blocks of protein and play a crucial role in numerous physiological functions. Dates contain a wide range of amino acids, both essential and non-essential.

Essential Amino Acids

- **Lysine:** Important for protein synthesis, strengthening the immune system and bone health.
- **Leucine:** Promotes muscle growth and cell regeneration.
- **Isoleucine:** Helps regulate blood sugar levels and muscle energy.
- **Valine:** Necessary for tissue repair and maintenance of muscle strength.

Dates therefore also contain branched-chain amino acids (BCAAs) and this explains why they bring significant benefits to athletes (professionals and amateurs) by promoting the regeneration of muscle cells and regulating muscle energy obtained from the consumption of sugars in the blood.

Non-essential amino acids

- **Arginine:** Supports cardiovascular function by improving blood circulation.
- **Glycine:** Promotes sleep and mental well-being by reducing oxidative stress.
- **Glutamic acid:** Essential for brain health and energy metabolism.

Chapter 10: Dates and Gestation, Childbirth and Puerperium

Dates, in the countries of origin, have always played an important role for pregnant women, during childbirth and in the postpartum period, thanks to their nutritional, energetic and medicinal properties. This chapter explores in detail the benefits of dates at these critical stages, with insights into uses in traditional and ancient medicine. Pregnancy and the puerperium are crucial phases in a woman's life, characterized by profound physiological, emotional and nutritional changes. During these times, adequate nutrient intake is essential for the mother's well-being and the baby's optimal development.

Physiological changes in pregnancy

1. Hormonal balance. From the moment of conception, there is an increase in levels of hormones such as:
- Progesterone: This hormone is essential for maintaining pregnancy. It is produced initially by the corpus luteum and later by the placenta. Progesterone has relaxing effects on smooth muscles, including those of the uterus, preventing premature contractions. It also promotes breast growth and fat metabolism.
- Estrogenic: estrogenic increases significantly during pregnancy and is responsible for numerous changes, including increasing blood flow to the uterus and stimulating the growth of breast tissues. Estrogenic also makes it easier to prepare the uterus for childbirth.
- HCG (Human Chorionic Gonadotropin): This hormone is produced by the placenta and is used as a marker in

pregnancy tests. It plays an important role in maintaining progesterone production in the early stages of pregnancy and supports the proper development of the foetus.

- Prolactin: This hormone stimulates milk production in the breast, preparing the mother for breastfeeding after childbirth.

2. The cardiovascular system undergoes numerous changes to meet the needs of the growing foetus. Some of the major adaptations include:

- Increased blood volume: During pregnancy, the blood volume in the mother increases by 30-50% to ensure adequate perfusion of the mother's organs and to meet the metabolic needs of the foetus. There is an increased need for absorbable iron.

- Increased heart rate: The mother's heart rate increases by about 10 to 20 beats per minute to accommodate the increase in blood volume.

- Changes to blood pressure: Blood pressure may experience a slight decrease in the first trimester due to dilated blood vessels, but it usually returns to pre-pregnancy levels by the end of pregnancy. In some women, however, gestational hypertension may develop.

- Increased cardiac output: Cardiac output (the amount of blood pumped by the heart in one minute) increases during pregnancy to ensure adequate oxygenation of maternal and foetal tissues.

3. The respiratory system is also subject to major changes to ensure that the mother and foetus receive sufficient oxygen. These changes include:

- Increased tidal volume: The volume of air entering the lungs with each breath increases during pregnancy, leading to improved oxygenation. This happens because of progesterone, which stimulates the respiratory centres in the brain.

- Increased breathing rate: Breathing rate tends to increase by about 2-3 breaths per minute.
- Chest expansion: The growing uterus puts pressure on the diaphragm, reducing the available chest space, but thanks to the relaxing action of progesterone, the ribcage expands and adapts.

4. The kidneys and urinary system undergo numerous changes to manage the increase in blood volume and substances to be eliminated. Some of the major changes include:

- Increased renal blood flow: Blood flow to the kidneys increases during pregnancy to ensure greater filtration of toxic substances and metabolic wastes.
- Increased urine output: As blood volume increases, the kidneys produce more urine to eliminate surplus fluid. However, the mother may be more prone to frequent urination, especially in the first and third trimesters, due to the pressure of the uterus on the kidneys and bladder.
- Changes in kidney function: Kidney function is optimized to eliminate waste products from both the mother and the foetus. Glomerular filtration increases by 40-50%, and this can lead to a slight reduction in creatinine levels in the blood.

5. Hormones cause several changes in the digestive system. Key changes include:

- Smooth muscle relaxation: Progesterone relaxes the smooth muscles of the gastrointestinal system, slowing down the transit of food and causing increased water retention in the stool, which can lead to constipation.

- Nausea and vomiting: In most women, the first trimester is characterized by nausea and vomiting, a phenomenon known as "morning sickness." This is likely caused by increased levels of HCG and estrogenic.
- Gastroesophageal acidity and reflux: Expansion of the uterus can compress the stomach, promoting acid reflux and indigestion, a common ailment during pregnancy.
6. Changes in the skin and hair, which are largely due to increased hormones and blood flow.
- Increased pigmentation: "Linea nigra" (a dark line that appears on the abdomen) and dark spots on the face, such as "melasma," are common during pregnancy and are caused by the hormone's estrogenic and progesterone.
- Increased hair growth: Due to hormonal changes, hair can grow faster and look thicker. However, after giving birth, many women notice temporary hair loss.
7. Basal metabolic rate: Calorie consumption increases to support the child's energy needs.
8. Body weight: Essential to support pregnancy, but an increase should be monitored to avoid complications.

Nutritional Needs in Pregnancy

The diet during pregnancy must be varied, balanced and rich in essential nutrients.

Macronutrients

- Proteins: Necessary for the growth of maternal and foetal tissues. An increase of about 10-15 grams per day is recommended
- Carbohydrates: Primary source of energy, they should make-up about 50-60% of daily calories. The overall caloric intake should increase by about 300-350 calories

per day during the second and third trimesters of pregnancy. In the first trimester, calorie increase is generally not necessary.

- Fat: During pregnancy, fat intake should account for about 25-35% of total daily calories. It is important to focus on healthy fats, such as monounsaturated and polyunsaturated fats, which are found in foods such as olive oil, avocados, fatty fish (e.g. salmon and mackerel), nuts and seeds. Omega-3 fatty acids (DHA and EPA) are essential for the brain development of the foetus.
- Fiber: Although fibre is not a macronutrient, it is essential during pregnancy. Fiber helps prevent constipation, which is a common problem during pregnancy due to hormonal and physical changes. A diet rich in dietary fibre (about 25-30 grams per day) is important for maintaining good digestion and intestinal health. The main sources of fibre are whole grains, legumes, fruits, and vegetables.

Micronutrients

- Folic acid: Crucial for preventing neural tube defects. A supplement of 200 micrograms per day (400 to 600) is recommended in the bibliography. Food sources: Green leafy vegetables, legumes, citrus fruits, fortified cereals, and folic acid supplements.
- Iron: A supplement of 10 mg. per day (from 18 to 28) is recommended in the bibliography. Essential to prevent maternal anaemia and ensure adequate oxygen transport to the foetus. Food sources include red meat, legumes, and leafy greens.
- Calcium: Important for the development of the child's bones and teeth. 1 gr/day. Food sources: Dairy products

(milk, yogurt, cheese), leafy greens, tofu, calcium-fortified drinks, and nuts.

- Vitamin D: Necessary for calcium absorption and bone health. Sun exposure and fortified foods are key sources. 600 IU/day. Food sources: Fatty fish (such as salmon and mackerel), eggs, milk, and fortified juices.
- Iodine: Essential for thyroid function and neurological development of the foetus. 220 micrograms/day. Food sources: Iodized salt, fish, dairy products, eggs.
- Vitamin B12: Vitamin B12 is essential to produce red blood cells and the health of the nervous system. Supplementation is especially important for vegetarian or vegan women, as vitamin B12 is mainly found in animal-based foods. During pregnancy, the recommended intake of vitamin B12 is 2.6 micrograms per day. Food sources: Meat, fish, eggs, dairy, and foods fortified with vitamin B12.
- Vitamin A: Vitamin A is crucial for the proper development of the foetus' visual system, immune system, and nervous system. However, it is important not to overdo it with your vitamin A intake, as too high doses can be harmful to the foetus. Daily requirement: The recommended intake of vitamin A during pregnancy is 770 micrograms of retinol equivalent per day. Food sources: Carrots, sweet potatoes, spinach, kale, and other orange or green vegetables, as well as liver (but in limited amounts).
- Zinc: Zinc is essential for cell growth and development, immune function, and DNA synthesis. Daily requirement: During pregnancy, women should take about 11 milligrams of zinc per day. Food sources: Red meat,

poultry, fish, legumes, pumpkin seeds, nuts, and whole grains.

- Omega-3 Fatty Acids (DHA): Omega-3 fatty acids are crucial for the development of the fetus' brain and eyes, especially DHA (docosahexaenoic acid). Daily requirements: Although there is no specific recommendation for omega-3 intake during pregnancy, it is suggested to consume 200-300 milligrams of DHA per day. Food sources: Fatty fish (such as salmon and mackerel), walnuts, flaxseed, and seaweed oil.

Common Nutritional Problems in Pregnancy

- **Nausea and vomiting**: These can impair nutritional intake. Practical solutions include small, frequent meals and ginger intake.
- **Iron deficiency anaemia**: Common due to increased blood requirements. It can be managed with iron supplements.
- **Gestational diabetes**: Requires a low glycaemic index diet and medical monitoring.
- **Excessive weight gain**: It can lead to obstetric complications. Personalized nutritional counselling can help.

Nutrition in the Puerperium

The puerperium is the postpartum period in which the mother's body recovers from the transformations of pregnancy. Nutritional needs continue to be high, especially for breastfeeding women.

Nutritional needs in lactation

- Calories: Breastfeeding requires about 500 extra calories per day.
- Proteins: Essential to produce breast milk.
- Fluids: Proper hydration is crucial to support milk production.
- Vitamins and minerals: The intake of calcium, iron, vitamin D and omega-3 remains a priority.

Common Nutritional Problems in the Puerperium

- Iron deficiency: Due to blood loss during childbirth. It can be prevented with a diet rich in iron and supplements if necessary.
- Fatigue and tiredness: A balanced diet helps to improve energy and support recovery.
- Rapid weight loss: It can impair milk production and overall health. Gradual weight loss is recommended.

Plan nutritious and simple meals to cope with limited time.
- Supplement your diet with foods rich in key nutrients such as fruits, vegetables, lean proteins, and whole grains.
- Avoid restrictive diets, especially during breastfeeding.

Pregnancy and the puerperium represent periods of great change that require special attention to nutrition. A balanced diet, accompanied by adequate medical and nutritional support, is essential for the health of mother and baby.

Benefits of Dates for Pregnant Women

Energy and Nutrition

- As already highlighted, during pregnancy, energy and nutrient requirements increase significantly. Dates are a natural source of immediate energy due to their high content of natural sugars (glucose and fructose) and essential nutrients.
- Iron: Essential for preventing anaemia, a common problem in pregnancy. Dates help maintain healthy haemoglobin levels.

- Calcium and Magnesium: Essential for the bone development of the foetus and to prevent muscle cramps in the mother.
- Fiber: They help regulate intestinal transit and prevent constipation, a common ailment during pregnancy.
- Folic acid: Although present in modest amounts, the consumption of dates can be a natural source and contribute to the prevention of neural malformations in the foetus.

Hormonal balance

- Dates contain natural compounds that can positively influence hormonal balance:
- **Uterine stimulation:** Some studies indicate that dates can help prepare the uterus for childbirth, thanks to the presence of compounds like oxytocin, the hormone that facilitates contractions.

Dates and Childbirth

Ease of Labor

- One of the most famous references to the use of dates during childbirth is found in the Qur'an (Sura of Mary, 19:25): *"And shake the trunk of the palm tree towards you: it will cause fresh, ripe dates to fall on you. Eat, drink, and comfort your heart."*
- This passage tells that Mary, the mother of Jesus, found comfort and strength by consuming dates during labour. This symbolic example is also reflected in the scientifically documented benefits.

Scientific evidence

1. A study published in the *Journal of Obstetrics and Gynaecology* found that consuming dates in the last weeks of pregnancy reduced the duration of labour and decreased the need for medical interventions.
2. Dates promote:
3. Natural uterine contractions: Stimulate the release of endogenous oxytocin.
4. Faster cervical dilation.

Traditional Practice

In many cultures in the Middle East and North Africa, traditional midwives gave dates to women in labour to provide energy and facilitate childbirth. This natural remedy was often combined with honey or ghee to strengthen its effects.

1. **Energy Recovery**
   - The postpartum period requires rapid physical recovery. Dates, with their simple sugar content, provide immediate energy without overloading the digestive system.
   - **Iron reconstitution:** Their iron content helps restore haemoglobin levels lost during childbirth.
   - **Lactation support:** It is believed that dates can promote breast milk production due to their combination of nutrients.

2. **Anti-inflammatory and healing properties**
   - Bioactive compounds in dates, such as flavonoids and polyphenols, reduce inflammation and speed up the wound healing process, including any stitches after childbirth.

Uses in Traditional and Ancient Medicine

Ayurvedic Medicine

Dates, called *khajoor*, are considered a natural tonic to strengthen women after childbirth. They were often prepared in the form of spiced milk with turmeric, ginger and cardamom.

North African Remedies

- **Date paste:** A date paste mixed with honey and ghee was given to mothers to speed up healing and improve mood.
- **Decoctions:** Date seeds were boiled to make a tea that relieved postpartum pain.

Ancient China

Chinese women included red dates (like traditional dates) in the postpartum diet to strengthen blood and improve vital energy (*qi*).

Traditional and Modern Recipes for Pregnant and Postpartum Women

Date Milk

Ingredients: 5 Medjool dates, 1 cup of milk (also vegetable), a pinch of cinnamon.

- **Procedure:** Blend the dates with warm milk and add cinnamon. Drink in the morning for energy.
- **Benefits:** Provides immediate energy and improves the quality of breast milk.

Energy Pasta with Dates

Ingredients: Dates, walnuts, sesame seeds, honey.

- **Procedure:** Blend the dates with walnuts and sesame seeds. Add honey to obtain a creamy paste.
- **Use:** One tablespoon a day to improve physical recovery.

Date Seed Infusion

Ingredients: Date seeds, water, ginger.

- **Procedure:** Boil date seeds with ginger for 20 minutes. Filter and drink.
- **Benefits:** Reduces uterine inflammation and promotes recovery.

Contraindications and Precautions

1. **Excess sugar:** Women with gestational diabetes should consume dates in moderation and under medical supervision.
2. **Allergies:** Although rare, some people may be allergic to dates.
3. **Portion balance:** Despite the benefits, it is important not to overeat to avoid too high a calorie intake.

Dates are an extraordinary food for pregnant women, during childbirth and in the puerperium. Their nutritional and medicinal properties, combined with the centuries-old traditions of ancient cultures, offer a natural approach to supporting maternal health. Consciously integrating them into the diet can promote a more serene and healthy motherhood experience, rooted in the wisdom of nature and tradition.

Chapter 11: The Use of Dates in Sport

Dates, thanks to their nutritional profile rich in natural sugars, minerals and amino acids, have been used for centuries as a source of energy and physical endurance. This chapter explores how dates are used in modern and traditional sport and tells how they were used in sports competitions and competitions in ancient times and among Arab and African peoples.

Properties of Sports Dates

Immediate Energy Source

Dates are rich in simple carbohydrates, mainly glucose and fructose, which are quickly metabolized by the body to provide immediate energy. This makes them ideal:

1. **Before exercise:** For a quick energy supply.
2. **During intense physical activity: As a** quick and easily digestible snack.
3. **After training:** To promote muscle recovery thanks to the combination of carbohydrates and amino acids.

Minerals for Recovery

1. **Potassium:** Helps prevent muscle cramps and promotes electrolyte balance.
2. **Magnesium:** Supports energy metabolism and muscle function.
3. **Iron:** Contributes to the production of red blood cells, improving muscle oxygenation.

Amino Acids for Regeneration

The amino acids found in dates, such as leucine and isoleucine, promote muscle tissue repair and protein synthesis, which is essential for endurance or strength athletes.

Use of Dates in Modern Sport

Natural Supplement

Dates are often preferred to artificial snacks due to their natural nutrient content. The following are used:

- **As energy bars:** Prepare with dates, oats and seeds.
- **As sports drinks:** Date smoothies with almond milk or coconut water.

Benefits for Endurance Athletes

- Runners, cyclists and swimmers use dates to quickly replenish glycogen stores during and after exercise.
- The combination of natural sugars and Fiber ensures a stable release of energy, avoiding glycaemic peaks.

Post-workout recovery

Due to the carbohydrate and potassium content, dates are great for restoring energy and balancing electrolytes lost through sweat.

Use of Dates in Sport in Antiquity

Arab peoples

Arab peoples used dates as their main food to sustain physical competition and endurance in the harsh desert conditions.

- **Running races:** During long-distance runs, runners used to consume dried dates to maintain energy.
- **Desert Knights:** Arabian warriors and horsemen, often engaged in equestrian competitions or simulated battles, carried dates as a supply to sustain long hours of physical exertion.

Specific Traditions

- **Date and camel milk blends:** Consider an ideal energy drink for athletes.
- **Dates and honey:** Used to make concentrated pasta to be consumed before races or long trips.

African peoples

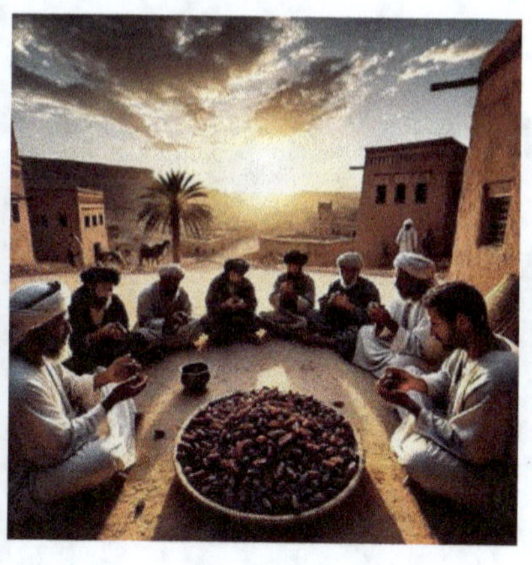

Traditional wrestling competitions: In some regions of North Africa, dates were consumed by wrestlers to increase strength and endurance.

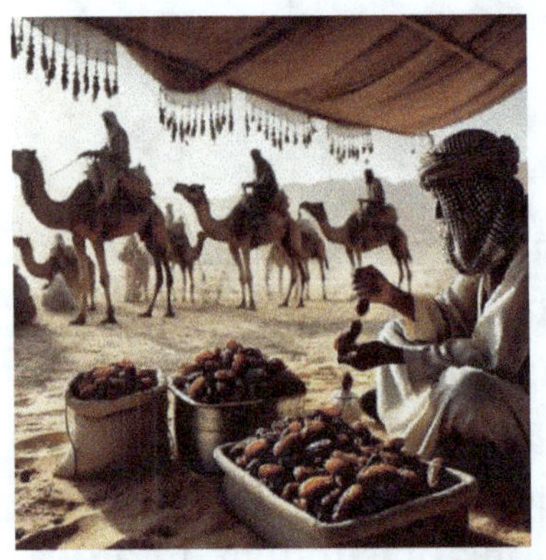

Travelers and athletes: Caravanners who participated in camel races consumed dates for energy and natural hydration.

Competitions of Antiquity

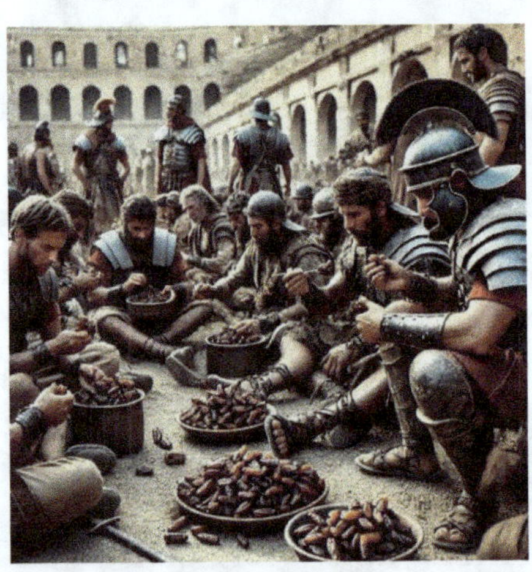

In the Roman Empire, influenced by contacts with the Middle East and North Africa, gladiators and soldiers consumed dates as a source of energy before fighting.

Stories and Legends about the Use of Dates in Sport

The Desert Race

A Bedouin legend tells of an epic competition between two tribes

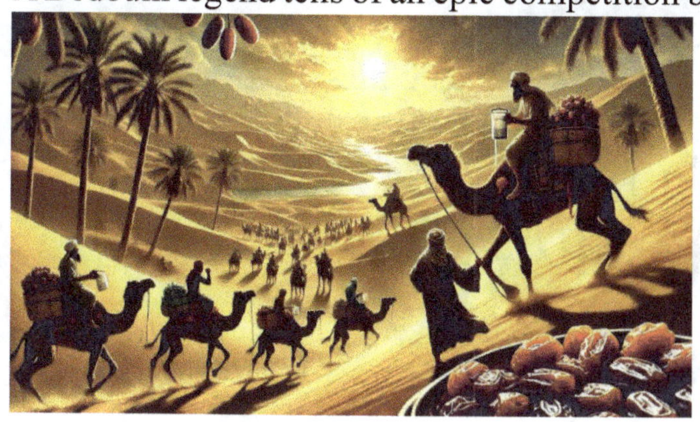

who had to cross the desert to reach an oasis. The participants, equipped with dates and camel milk, managed to complete the race despite the extreme conditions. It is said that those who consumed ripe Medjool dates had more strength and endurance.

The energy of Arab warriors

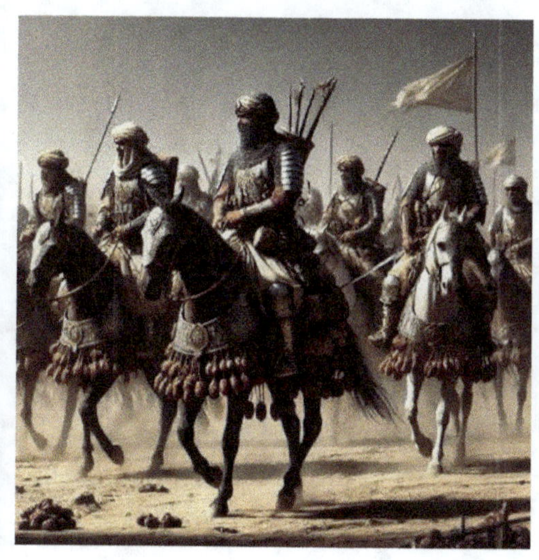

According to a popular story, Saladin's Arab knights during the Crusades always carried dried dates in their saddlebags, considering them an indispensable source of strength for battles and competitions of skill.

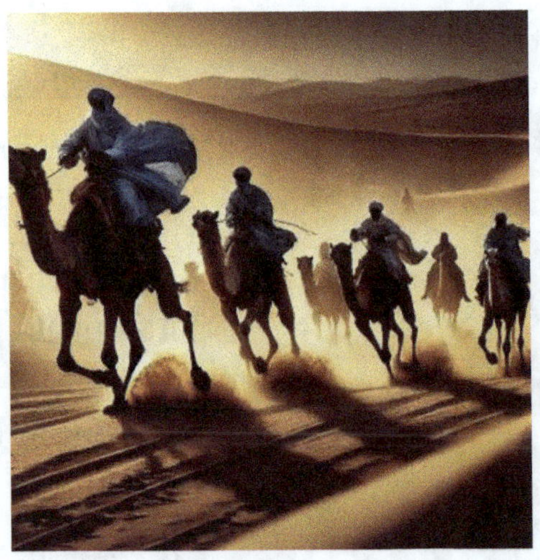

The Tuaregs, known as the "blue men of the desert," used dates as their only food during long runs across the Sahara. It was said that a single date could sustain a man for an entire day, thanks to its calorie and nutrient content.

Recipes for Athletes based on Dates

Date Energy Bars

Ingredients: Dates, walnuts, chia seeds, oatmeal, peanut butter.

- **Procedure:** Blend all the ingredients, roll out the dough and let it set in the refrigerator. Cut into bars.
- **Benefit:** Immediate energy, rich in carbohydrates and healthy fats.

Date Hydration Drink

Ingredients: 5 dates, 500 ml of water, a pinch of pink salt, lemon juice.

- **Procedure:** Allow the dates to soak in water overnight, then blend. Add salt and lemon.
- **Benefit:** Restores electrolytes lost during training.

Pre-Workout Smoothie

Ingredients: 4 dates, a banana, almond milk, cocoa powder.

- **Procedure:** Blend all the ingredients until creamy.
- **Benefit:** Gradual energy release, suitable for endurance sports.

Indications and Contraindications

Directions

- **Endurance sports:** Perfect for runners, cyclists and swimmers thanks to the fast energy release.
- **Muscle recovery:** Ideal for replenishing glycogen and minerals after intense efforts.

Contraindications

- **Calorie excess:** Athletes in the weight control phase must monitor their consumption of dates.
- **Diabetes or insulin resistance:** Natural sugars can cause blood sugar spikes if not balanced with protein or Fiber.

Dates are an ideal food for athletes, thanks to their unique nutritional profile that combines natural sugars, essential minerals and amino acids. In ancient times, peoples such as the Arabs and Africans used them to face competitions and physical challenges, appreciating their ability to provide energy and endurance in extreme conditions. Today, rediscovering dates in sport means embracing a thousand-year-old tradition and harnessing a natural resource to improve athletic performance and recovery.

Chapter 12: A Thousand-Year Fruit between Tradition and Science

Dates are much more than just a food: they represent a deep link between tradition, culture and modern science. From palm trees that soar through the desert as symbols of resilience and abundance, to their sweet and nutritious fruits, dates have nourished humanity for millennia, accompanying civilizations through times of prosperity and challenge.

A Gift from Nature

The date palm (*Phoenix dactylifera*) has been called the "tree of life" for its many uses. Every part of the plant, from the trunk to the fruits, is a testament to how nature offers complete resources for human sustenance. Dates are not just a source of food, but a gift that nourishes the body, comforts the soul, and supports health.

The Meeting of History and Modernity

The journey of dates in this book has led us:

1. **From ancient history**, where dates were a symbol of fertility and abundance, consumed by pharaohs, merchants and warriors.
2. **To religious traditions**, where they appear as blessed food in the Qur'an and in many spiritual practices.
3. **To modern science**, which has confirmed what ancient cultures intuitively knew: dates are a functional food, rich in therapeutic properties.

The Balance of Nutrition

Dates demonstrate how a natural food can meet a wide range of needs:

1.   **Immediate energy:** Thanks to natural sugars, essential for athletes and people looking for quick energy.
2.   **Health support:** Rich in fibres, minerals, amino acids, and antioxidants, they help the body fight chronic diseases, reduce inflammation, and improve digestion.
3.   **Specific benefits:** From supporting pregnant women to protecting against oxidative stress and inflammation, dates prove to be a valuable ally at different stages of life.

A Bridge Between Culture and Science

Stories handed down from generation to generation, like the traditional remedies of Arab and African peoples, are intertwined with modern science. This synergy demonstrates that empirical knowledge of ancient cultures can be confirmed and enriched by scientific research, reinforcing the importance of respecting and preserving traditions.

The Future of Dates

In a world that is increasingly looking towards sustainable diets and functional foods, dates offer a model of balance between environmental sustainability and health. Date palms grow in arid soils, transforming the desert into an oasis of life and prosperity. Their low environmental impact, combined with the growing demand for nutritious and natural foods, makes them protagonists of the diet of the future.

Prospects:

1. **Agricultural innovations:** Improved cultivation techniques to optimize the yield of date palms, reducing the use of resources.
2. **Pharmaceutical applications:** Date extracts could be used to develop new drugs or supplements against chronic diseases.
3. **Global expansion:** The accessibility of dates as a universal ingredient makes them suitable for a wide range of cuisines and eating habits.

6. An Invitation to Discovery

Dates are not just a food of the past or present: they are a symbol of how food can bring people together, heal the body and nourish the spirit. This book is an invitation to rediscover dates, not only as food, but as a treasure trove of cultural and scientific wisdom. Whether it's for a traditional recipe, a modern energy bar or a natural remedy, dates teach us that the simplicity of nature can offer extraordinary solutions.

In every date there is a story, an energy, and a fragment of that deep connection between man and nature that we must learn to cherish.

Bibliography

History of Date Palms

- Abdelhafiz, A. T., & Muhamad, J. A. (2008). *Midwives' knowledge, attitudes and practices towards the use of dates (Phoenix dactylifera) during labour.* Journal of Midwifery & Women's Health, 53(6), 546-550.
- Beech, M., 2003. Archaeobotanical Evidence for Early Date Consumption in the Arabian Gulf, in: The date Palm e from Traditional Resource to Green Wealth. The Emirates Center for Strategic Studies and Research, Abu Dhabi, pp. 11e31.
- Hawting, G. R. (2003). *The Idea of Idolatry and the Emergence of Islam: From Polemic to History*. Cambridge University Press.
- Munier, P. (1973). *Le palmier-dattier*. Maisonneuve & Larose.
- Murphy, C., & Fuller, D. Q. (2017). "The transition to agriculture in Arabia: Assessing the evidence from the domestication of the date palm (Phoenix dactylifera L.)." *Journal of Arid Environments*, 137, 42-54.
- Nevo, Y. (1991). "Religious Symbolism in Early Islam." *Bulletin of the School of Oriental and African Studies*, 54(3), 395-411.
- Terral, J.-F., et al. (2012). "Insights into the historical biogeography of the date palm (Phoenix dactylifera L.) using geometric morphometrics of modern and ancient seeds." *Journal of Biogeography*, 39(5), 929-941.
- Tengberg, M. (2012). "Beginnings and early history of date palm garden cultivation in the Middle East. *Journal of Arid Environments*, 86, 139-147.
- Vicino Oriente antico. Agricoltura e irrigazione." *Treccani - Storia della Scienza.*
- Zohary, D., & Hopf, M. (2000). *Domestication of Plants in the Old World*. Oxford University Press.

Nutritional Properties of Dates

- Al-Shahib, W., & Marshall, R. J. (2003). *The fruit of the date palm: its possible use as the best food for the future.* International Journal of Food Sciences and Nutrition, 54(4), 247-259.
- Vayalil, P. K. (2012). *Date fruits (Phoenix dactylifera Linn): an emerging medicinal food.* Critical Reviews in Food Science and Nutrition, 52(3), 249-271.

Chemical and Pharmacological Properties

- Baliga, M. S., Baliga, B. R. V., Kandathil, S. M., Bhat, H. P., & Vayalil, P. K. (2011). *A review of the chemistry and pharmacology of the date fruits (Phoenix dactylifera L.).* Food Research International, 44(7), 1812-1822.
- Cowan, M. M. (1999). Plant products as antimicrobial agents. *Clinical Microbiology Reviews*, 12(4), 564-582. https://doi.org/10.1128/CMR.12.4.564
- Cushnie, T. T., & Lamb, A. J. (2011). Recent advances in understanding the antibacterial properties of flavonoids and related polyphenols. *International Journal of Antimicrobial Agents*, 38(2), 99-107. https://doi.org/10.1016/j.ijantimicag.2011.02.014.
- Daglia, M. (2012). Polyphenols as antimicrobial agents. *Current Opinion in Biotechnology*, 23(2), 174-181. https://doi.org/10.1016/j.copbio.2011.08.005
- Okuda, T., & Ito, H. (2011). Tannins and related polyphenols: Perspectives for their pharmacological properties. *Journal of Natural Products*, 74(3), 501-515. https://doi.org/10.1021/np100924u.
- Scalbert, A. (1991). Antimicrobial properties of tannins. *Phytochemistry*, 30(12), 3875-3883. https://doi.org/10.1016/0031-9422(91)83426-L

Antioxidant and Anti-Inflammatory Properties

- Allaith, A. A. A. (2008). *Antioxidant activity of Bahraini date palm (Phoenix dactylifera L.) fruit of various cultivars*. International Journal of Food Science & Technology, 43(6), 1033-1040.
- Bhattacharya, S. (2014). Reactive oxygen species and cellular defense system. *Free Radical Biology and Medicine*, 76, 133-152. https://doi.org/10.1016/j.freeradbiomed.2014.08.032
- Bettaieb, I., Kilani, A., Ben Othman, K., Benabderrahim, M.A., Elfalleh, W., 2023. Phenolic profile, sugar composition, and antioxidant capacities of some common date palm (Phoenix dactylifera L.) cultivars as a potential nutraceutical and functional food ingredients. J. Food Qual.
- Calder, P. C. (2020). Nutrition, immunity and COVID-19. *BMJ Nutrition, Prevention & Health*, 3(1), 74-92. https://doi.org/10.1136/bmjnph-2020-000085
- Hossam S. El-Beltagi, Syed Tanveer Shah, Heba I. Mohamed, Nabeel Alam, Muhammad Sajid, Ayesha Khan, Abdul Basit, 2023. Physiological response, phytochemicals, antioxidant, and enzymatic activity of date palm (Phoenix dactylifera L.) cultivated under different storage time, harvesting Stages, and temperatures. Saudi Journal of Biological Sciences.
- Libby, P. (2002). Inflammation in atherosclerosis. *Nature*, 420(6917), 868-874. https://doi.org/10.1038/nature01323
- Mahomoodally, M.F., Khadaroo, S.K., Hosenally, M., Zengin, G., Rebezov, M., Ali Shariati, M., Khalid, A., Abdalla, A.N., Algarni, A.S., Simal-Gandara, J., 2023. Nutritional, medicinal and functional properties of different parts of the date palm and its fruit (Phoenix dactylifera L.) – A systematic review. Crit. Rev. Food Sci. Nut
- Mandel, S., & Youdim, M. B. (2004). Catechin polyphenols: Neurodegeneration and neuroprotection in neurodegenerative diseases. *Free Radical Biology and Medicine*, 37(3), 304-317. https://doi.org/10.1016/j.freeradbiomed.2004.04.012
- Middleton, E., Jr., et al. (2000). The effects of plant flavonoids on mammalian cells: Implications for inflammation, heart disease, and cancer. *Pharmacological Reviews*, 52(4), 673-751. https://doi.org/10.1124/pr.52.4.673

- Pan, M. H., Lai, C. S., & Ho, C. T. (2010). Anti-inflammatory activity of natural dietary flavonoids. *Food & Function*, 1(1), 15-31. https://doi.org/10.1039/C0FO00103A
- Santos, C. N., et al. (2010). Polyphenols and neuroprotection: Impact on brain function. *Antioxidants & Redox Signaling*, 13(3), 343-394. https://doi.org/10.1089/ars.2009.3027
- Spencer, J. P. E. (2010). The impact of fruit flavonoids on memory and cognition. *British Journal of Nutrition*, 104(S3), S40-S47. https://doi.org/10.1017/S0007114510003934
- Scholey, A., & Owen, L. (2013). Effects of polyphenols on cognitive function in humans: A review of recent clinical trials. *Nutrition*, 29(7-8), 741-747. https://doi.org/10.1016/j.nut.2012.11.004
- Vauzour, D., et al. (2008). The neuroprotective potential of flavonoids: A multiplicity of effects. *Genes & Nutrition*, 3(3-4), 115-126. https://doi.org/10.1007/s12263-008-0091-4

Amino Acids and Sugars in Dates

- Al-Farsi, M., & Lee, C. Y. (2008). *Nutritional and functional properties of dates: a review*. Critical Reviews in Food Science and Nutrition, 48(10), 877-887.

Use of Dates in Gestation, Childbirth and Postpartum Women

- Al-Kuran O, Al-Mehaisen L, Bawadi H, Beitawi S, Amarin Z. The effect of late pregnancy consumption of date fruit on labour and delivery. *J Obstet Gynaecol*. 2011;31(1)
- Allen, L. H. "Multiple micronutrients in pregnancy and lactation: an overview." American Journal of Clinical Nutrition, 2005.
- American College of Obstetricians and Gynecologists. "Nutrition During Pregnancy." ACOG, 2021
- Institute of Medicine. "Nutrition During Pregnancy: Part I, Weight Gain; Part II, Nutrient Supplements." National Academies Press, 1990.

- Khadivzadeh T, Ghabel M. Complementary and alternative medicine use in pregnancy in Mashhad, Iran, 2007–8. *Iran J Nurs Midwifery Res.* 2012;17(4):263–269 PMID: 23833624.
- Koletzko, B., et al. "Dietary fat intakes for pregnant and lactating women." British Journal of Nutrition, 2007.
- Kordi M, Meybodi FA, Tara F, Fakari FR, Nemati M, Shakeri M. Effect of dates in late pregnancy on the duration of labor in nulliparous women. *Iran J Nurs Midwifery Res.* 2017;22(5):383–387. https://doi.org/10.4103/ijnmr.IJNMR_213_15 PMID: 29033994.
- Kordi, M., & Meybodi, F. A. (2014). *The effect of late-pregnancy consumption of date fruit on labor and delivery.* Journal of Midwifery and Reproductive Health, 2(3), 150-156.
- Kordi M, Aghaei Meybodi F, Tara F, Nemati M, Shakeri MT. The effect of latepregnancy consumption of date fruit on cervical ripening in nulliparous women. *J Midwif Rep Health.* 2014;2(3):150–156. https://doi.org/10.22038/jmrh.2014.2772.
- Razali N, Mohd Nahwari SH, Sulaiman S, Hassan J. Date fruit consumption at term: Effect on length of gestation, labour and delivery. *J Obstet Gynaecol.* 2017;37(5):595–600. https://doi.org/10.1080/01443615.2017 PMID: 28286995.
- Sendra E, Pratamaningtyas S, Panggayuh A. Effect of date palm (Phoenix dactylifera) consumption against the increase in hemoglobin levels in the second trimester of pregnant women in Puskesmas Ngadiluwih, Kediri. *J Ilmu Kesehat.* 2016;5(1):96–104.
- World Health Organization. "Guideline: Daily Iron and Folic Acid Supplementation in Pregnant Women." WHO, 2012.

Use of Dates in Sport

- Ahmed, T., et al. (2020). "Comparative effects of dates and commercial energy gels on athletic performance." *Journal of Sports Science & Medicine*, 19(3), 456-464.
- Ali, A., & Al-Kindi, Y. S. (2004). *Chemical composition and glycemic index of three varieties of Omani dates.* International Journal of Food Sciences and Nutrition, 55(6), 463-470.

- Ali, M. A., et al. (2016). "Date fruit consumption enhances endurance performance in long-distance runners." *Nutrients*, 8(6), 323.
- Al-Shahib, W., & Marshall, R. J. (2003). "The fruit of the date palm: Its possible use as the best food for the future" *International Journal of Food Sciences and Nutrition*, 54(4), 247-259.
- Rahmani, A. H., et al. (2014). "Nutritional aspects and health benefits of dates: A review." *Journal of Food Science and Technology*, 51(3), 661-670.

Marco Delledonne has twenty years of experience as an adjunct professor of Hygiene and Risk Analysis in the Degree Courses in Food Science and Technology of the Catholic University of the Sacred Heart.

He was Director of the Department of Public Health and the Food Safety Program of the Piacenza Health Authority and played the role of Competent Authority for Food and Chemical Safety of the Province of Piacenza.

He is the author of books on food safety and food labelling issues and has published many popular articles on food contamination issues in medical and trade journals.

He is an author and lecturer in refresher courses for Medical and Health Personnel, accredited by the Ministry of Health on food risk and food contamination issues.

He has participated, as a speaker on food safety issues, in several scientific conferences.

Since 2023 he has been the owner of a professional consulting firm in the field of Public Health and Food Safety.